The CADET NURSE CORPS *in* ARIZONA

ELSIE M. SZECSY
foreword by Richard Carmona

The CADET NURSE CORPS *in* ARIZONA

A History of Service

THE History PRESS

Published by The History Press
Charleston, SC
www.historypress.net

Front cover: Courtesy of the Sisters of St. Joseph of Carondelet, Los Angeles Province.

First published 2016

Manufactured in the United States

ISBN 978.1.46711.825.5

Library of Congress Control Number: 2015957665

Notice: The information in this book is true and complete to the best of our knowledge. It is offered without guarantee on the part of the author or The History Press. The author and The History Press disclaim all liability in connection with the use of this book.

I dedicate this book to all cadet nurses, for your tireless service, and to your families and friends who help keep this story alive. Proceeds from the sale of this book will be used to support the uscadetnurse.org website.

CONTENTS

FOREWORD

As the seventeenth surgeon general of the United States and a former registered nurse, I am elated that this wonderful and unique story of the selfless service of the U.S. Cadet Nurse Corps is finally receiving its long-overdue recognition.

This thoughtful book reveals an essential but forgotten part of America's wartime history. The Cadet Nurse Corps was a uniformed service of the United States that became part of the U.S. Public Health Service to answer the call to duty for registered nurses who were desperately needed during World War II. Aside from the essential nursing services these 124,000 nurses provided across the nation, they were also innovators and agents of change. The program was fully integrated and discrimination by race, ethnicity and marital status was prohibited. The nation's first and only accredited School of Nursing for Native Americans contributed to this endeavor as well. Minority participation was the norm and preceded any national formal minority student initiatives by decades. This program also prevented the collapse of our nation's healthcare delivery system during World War II and prevented a "draft" for nurses.

These nurses were part of what is now called the "Greatest Generation." As Rosie the Riveter and many other women did, these nurses stepped up, subordinated their personal interests and their families to serve selflessly, humbly and anonymously when the nation needed them most. At the end of the war, these great Americans quietly returned to their communities with no recognition but with the pride of having served in uniform and having made a huge difference to the health of the nation.

Make no mistake, although technically not considered veterans, these nurses are veterans just like all of us who have served when our nation called.

My hope is that this book will highlight and memorialize their exemplary service and that our nation will finally recognize the remaining nurses as heroes who served when needed. In doing so, they created many best practices that benefitted future nursing education.

RICHARD H. CARMONA, MD, MPH, FACS
Seventeenth Surgeon General of the United States

PREFACE

About five years ago, while going through some family heirlooms, I stumbled across my mother's nurse's cap and a couple of U.S. Cadet Nurse Corps sleeve patches. I had a faint recollection that my mother was a cadet nurse; she entered nursing school in a public hospital in Westchester County, New York, in the fall of 1943 and graduated in 1946. On a whim, since the computer was on and I was at my desk, I googled U.S. Cadet Nurse Corps and stumbled across a number of references, including an article in a local Massachusetts newspaper about a nurse interviewer with the Harvard Nurses' Health Study who had made a presentation about the U.S. Cadet Nurse Corps for a meeting of the Visiting Nurse Service somewhere in Massachusetts. Through her work as an interviewer, this woman learned that many of her respondents were cadet nurses. Since the article was recent, I thought that perhaps there was something important about cadet nurses, and I wanted to learn more. From that point, in October 2011, I was hooked.

I suspected that there was a possibility that cadet nurses all over the country were telling their stories to a local audience without knowing that they were not alone in telling the story. My first task, then, was to scour the Internet for additional information about the U.S. Cadet Nurse Corps. What I suspected was, indeed, the case. That research resulted in the uscadetnurse.org website, which I continue to curate, as well as a Facebook page to connect cadet nurses with one another. Both collect all sorts of information about the U.S. Cadet Nurse Corps, its history as the first federally funded education program for women, news items and scholarship.

Most important is that these two online tools collect the stories of cadet nurses, most now in their nineties, in their own words; these resources have also attracted and engaged family members and friends who want to know more about cadet nurses and what they were doing during and after World War II.

Next, as word got around at work, I learned that a professor of nursing at my university had conducted oral history interviews with twenty-five cadet nurses who were in Arizona during the 1980s. The transcripts of these interviews were archived in my university's library. What an opportunity! I read them and was thoroughly impressed by these women's observations and experiences and how timeless their accounts were. Many of the themes I was picking up through anecdotal data online on uscadetnurse.org were similar to the observations of these twenty-five women in the 1980s.

Within a year, another fortuitous coincidence happened. The National Archives, in partnership with ancestry.com, made the membership cards of cadet nurses available online. I was excited by this prospect to conduct additional historical research, and with this new development, a research agenda was born.

My original plan was to focus on my mother's experience in the state of New York. Now that membership card data was available, that would make for a wonderful study of cadet nurses and honor my mother's memory. When I saw there were over one hundred schools of nursing in New York, I thought twice about proceeding. I decided to find out about my adopted home state of Arizona and was pleasantly surprised to find out that there were only five participating schools of nursing in the U.S. Cadet Nurse Corps here. That number of schools was certainly on a scale that I could handle on my own and on the fringes of my life in the place where I am now planted. I have found that I am still honoring my mother's memory through this work and have, through this project, grown new roots in Arizona.

Now, I'd like to make some disclosures. I am not a nurse; I am an educator. Commenting on the quality of the contents of nurse curricula is outside my scope because I am not a nurse or nurse educator. So this book is not about nurse education curriculum development, training practices or the qualifications of nursing faculty. I approached the U.S. Cadet Nurse Corps simply as a historical phenomenon; it was a federally funded educational policy project with deep roots and far-reaching implications about which most people, I would argue, are largely unaware.

Neither am I a political scientist, sociologist or advocate. Despite the arguably correct assertion among many that cadet nurses have been inadequately recognized for their service during the war, the purpose of this book is not to advocate; its purpose is simply to educate. If some readers are moved by this book to share knowledge to inform others about this important program and group of women, then the book has served its purpose. I hope readers take away a clearer understanding about how instrumental women in the U.S. Cadet Nurse Corps were not only to Arizona and this nation during World War II but also to the nursing profession in the decades that followed. Perhaps equipped with this knowledge, readers will learn how to appropriately respect and recognize these volunteers and their legacy to our nation, the nursing profession and humanity.

This book is the beginning, I hope, of something much larger, as through this book I only scratch the surface of a profoundly rich topic.

ACKNOWLEDGEMENTS

This book grew out of a paper that was presented at the 2014 annual conference of the American Association for the History of Nursing in Hartford, Connecticut, and with the support of the School of Transborder Studies in the College of Liberal Arts and Sciences, Arizona State University, through a sabbatical. I am indebted to my colleagues at ASU, including Carlos Vélez-Ibáñez, Edward Escobar, Gayle Gullett, Francisco Lara-Valencia, Maria Luz Cruz Torres, Patricia Corona, Norma Valenzuela and Marta Sánchez, whose encouragement and insights contributed to an ever-improving narrative for this book.

I am also indebted to archivists who helped me locate critical information for this study: Christine Marin, academic professional emerita and archivist of the Chicano/a Research Collection and the Arizona Collection in the Department of Archives & Special Collections, Hayden Library at Arizona State University, pointed me to the oral history transcripts that Joyce Finch collected; she also introduced me to Sylvia Jiménez's story and Sylvia's family. ASU Libraries archivist Robert Spindler was also very instrumental in connecting me with other resources that contributed additional texture to this book's narrative. Diane Gallagher, nursing history and university archivist in the Howard Gotlieb Archive and Research Center at Boston University, connected me with Joyce Finch's 1988 presentation abstract in the American Association for the History of Nursing archives in residence at Boston University. I also appreciate the efforts of University of Arizona Health Sciences librarian Hannah Fischer, as well as Kathleen Scheppler and Bryan Nugent at the Banner-University Medical Center Medical Library for their assistance in connecting me with little-known information about Sage Memorial and Good Samaritan Hospital schools of nursing, respectively. I owe a similar debt of gratitude to Sister Patricia Rose Shanahan, CSJ, and Carol Smith, CSJ, at the Los Angeles Province of the Sisters of St. Joseph of Carondelet for information about Saint Mary's in Tucson and to Sister Madonna Marie Bolton, CSM, at the Saint Joseph's Medical Center, for her help in clarifying the involvement of the Sisters of Saint Joseph and the Sisters of Mercy in building those institutions. I would not have found this information without them.

To Shirley Harrow, RN, who introduced me to many cadet nurses and who is my coach, cheerleader and friend, I owe my deepest gratitude. To cadet nurse Thelma Robinson, RN, MS, go my heartfelt thanks for her generosity in making resources from her scholarship on cadet nurses available to enrich the content of this book. I am honored to know Thelma. Special thanks go to Josué González, esteemed colleague, mentor and friend, who shared my excitement with every discovery about the cadet nurses over the years. Their review of work leading up to this book resulted in an improved product.

I have been humbled by the contact I have had with cadet nurses and their brothers, sisters, sons and daughters, who have been most helpful in facilitating these connections. Thank you. To all of the cadet nurses who I have had the pleasure to meet in person, on the phone, through letters and via the uscadetnurse.org website and companion Facebook page over the past few years, you have all inspired me to continue learning.

To our nation's seventeenth surgeon general, Dr. Richard Carmona, thank you for your leadership in the U.S. Public Health Service. Thank you also for consenting to write the foreword for this book. It means so much to me. Your words help us see important details in this story more accurately.

I am also indebted to Megan Laddusaw, acquisitions editor at The History Press, who noticed my topic in the Arizona Humanities catalogue of speakers and who thought it good enough to invite me to write a book. I also owe thanks to Julia Turner, who edited the manuscript, as well as to the rest of the editorial and design teams at The History Press. Their efforts and creativity contributed to a well-designed publication and an as clearly written narrative as possible.

And finally, to Cadet Nurse Elsie Felicia Ulrich Szecsy, RN, words cannot express how much I have come to appreciate the true value of your investment in me, Mom. Though you did not train in Arizona, your heart has been and continues to be very much a part of me during this Arizona sojourn.

INTRODUCTION

The U.S. Cadet Nurse Corps, a federal program and innovation for its time, addressed a healthcare emergency during World War II—a shortage of nurses—and called for an end to discrimination by race, ethnicity or marital status. The corps' organizational structure was decentralized, which allowed for local control over how nurse training would be structured within the context of national nurse education standards. This development arose at a time when it was not uncommon for African American women to be denied admission to white nursing schools and when African American nursing schools did not always follow the same standard as nursing schools for white women. African American students attended separate nursing schools from white students. Little is known about the degree to which schools of nursing participating in the Cadet Nurse Corps actually admitted students regardless of race or ethnicity under the terms of the Nurse Training Act of 1943. Also unknown is how nurses of various races and ethnicities related with one another at work. The purpose of this book is to explore these and other questions in Arizona.

This book is divided into five chapters. In the first chapter, I give an overview of the history of this federally funded program's genesis from its introduction as a bill in Congress to its enactment as law in 1943. I also describe how the states, including Arizona, were involved in the recruitment of young women to serve in the Cadet Nurse Corps.

In the second chapter is a description of the environment in which Arizona cadet nurses found themselves when they were in training. The state of Arizona was rich with federally owned land, so there were many federally operated installations across the state, which drove the wartime economy and brought many people from places across the country and the globe, some willingly and some not so willingly.

The third chapter is devoted to the history of the five participating Arizona schools of nursing in the U.S. Cadet Nurse Corps program. In order to give the most complete impression possible to the reader, I discuss these schools' histories from their beginnings, which go as far back as 1910 in the Arizona Territory (Arizona achieved statehood in 1912).

The fourth chapter offers impressions of Arizona Cadet Nurses' experiences and is based primarily on two data sources. The first source is their membership card files, which provided insights into their life trajectories until their enlistment in the corps, as well as their success as nursing students and completion of their program of study. The second source was a collection of twenty-five oral history transcripts from interviews taken in the late 1980s with cadet nurses who had worked as nurses after World War II in Arizona. From these two and other data sources, such as cadet nurse obituaries, I highlight ten cadet nurses in the fifth chapter.

I raise questions about the program not only for our nation during World War II but also, and perhaps more importantly, in the decades that followed. I also draw tentative conclusions that this program had a profound effect on our nation's health, the process of professionalizing nursing and the status of women. In addition to these, I posit some deductions about women's leadership in Arizona, a leadership that spanned many decades throughout the twentieth century, including the World War II years, and crossed racial and ethnic boundaries.

This impressionistic exploration will describe many contributions of the program to social change both in the short term and over the span of decades. As a result of this exploration, additional questions about the interplay between federal policy and nurse education in these five uniquely situated Arizona hospital schools of nursing, as well as with other schools of nursing nationally, will emerge. Tentative connections between the nondiscrimination clause of the Nurse Training Act of 1943 and nurse education in Arizona will be proposed. Additional questions concerning the qualitative context for these connections before, during and after World War II will be raised.

Chapter 1

U.S. CADET NURSE CORPS LEGISLATION AND FEATURES

The nursing shortage during World War II was nothing new. A nursing shortage had existed since World War I. In order to address this problem, during the period between the world wars, efforts were made to professionalize nursing and to provide for a standardized curriculum. Also, a "separate but equal" approach had been the norm in nurse education. Before World War II, there were separate nurse training programs for white and African American students. However, there was no guarantee that the quality of these different programs was equivalent.

In the Goldmark Report,[1] commissioned by the Rockefeller Foundation in 1920, the authors found that nurse education was inadequate. They called for educational standards–based nursing education at colleges or universities and advanced degrees for nurse educators. Through this report, they also recommended a migration of nurse education from an apprenticeship model that suited the needs of hospitals to an academic model that equipped nurses for an expanded role in healthcare and education. As World War II began, there was already a shortage of nurses, and attempts were made to encourage young women to become nurses and to encourage older, inactive nurses to return to the profession. These efforts were not successful in easing the shortage. With this nursing shortage and the impending U.S. involvement in World War II, nurse educators across the country were eager to serve, but they also wanted to be sure that progress made in improving the curriculum and status of nursing was not eroded by the war effort.

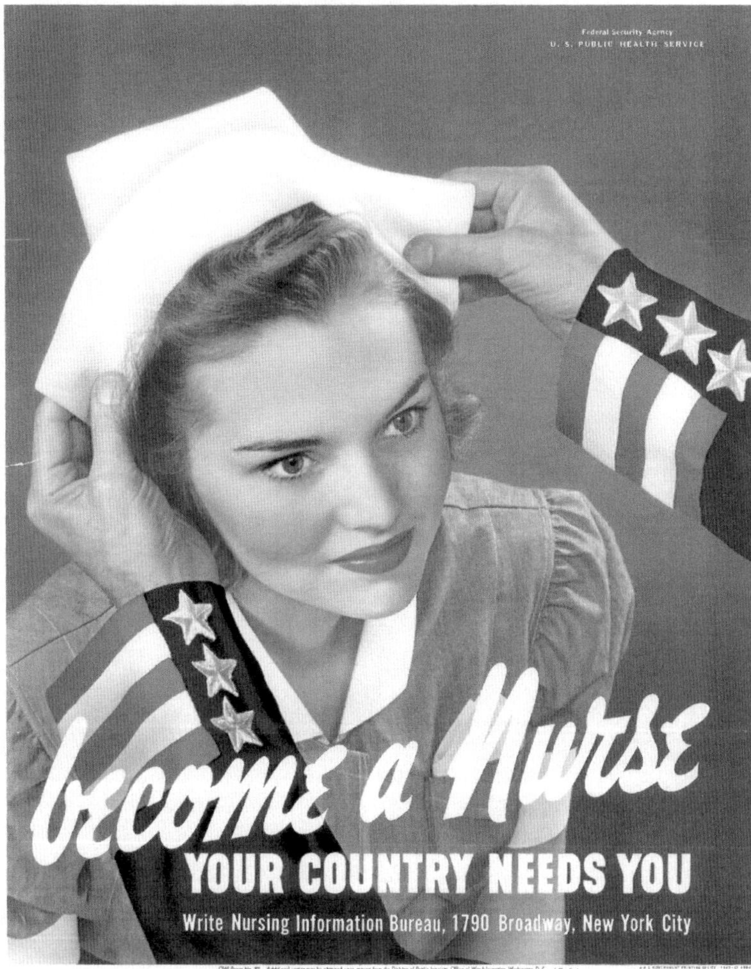
Federal Security Agency
U. S. PUBLIC HEALTH SERVICE
become a Nurse
YOUR COUNTRY NEEDS YOU
Write Nursing Information Bureau, 1790 Broadway, New York City

Created in 1942 by the American Nurses Association, Nurse Information Bureau, this poster shows a young woman receiving her nursing cap. A male (only the hands and sleeves are shown) is placing it on her head. He wears blue sleeves with a stars-and-stripes motif on the cuffs. The young woman wears a blue cotton uniform with a white collar, cuffs and pocket handkerchief. *University of North Texas Libraries, Government Documents Department.*

After the United States entered World War II, the need for military nurses quickly emptied hospitals of nurses, thus bringing on a stateside nursing shortage. To address this problem and to avoid a draft for nurses, Congress unanimously approved legislation that resulted in the establishment of the U.S. Cadet Nurse Corps.

In 1943, under the leadership of Representative Frances Payne Bolton of Ohio, Congress authorized the Nurse Training Act of 1943.[2] On June 15, 1943, President Franklin Delano Roosevelt enacted the law, which was also known as the Bolton Act. The U.S. Cadet Nurse Corps started operation on July 1, 1943. The program was administered by the U.S.

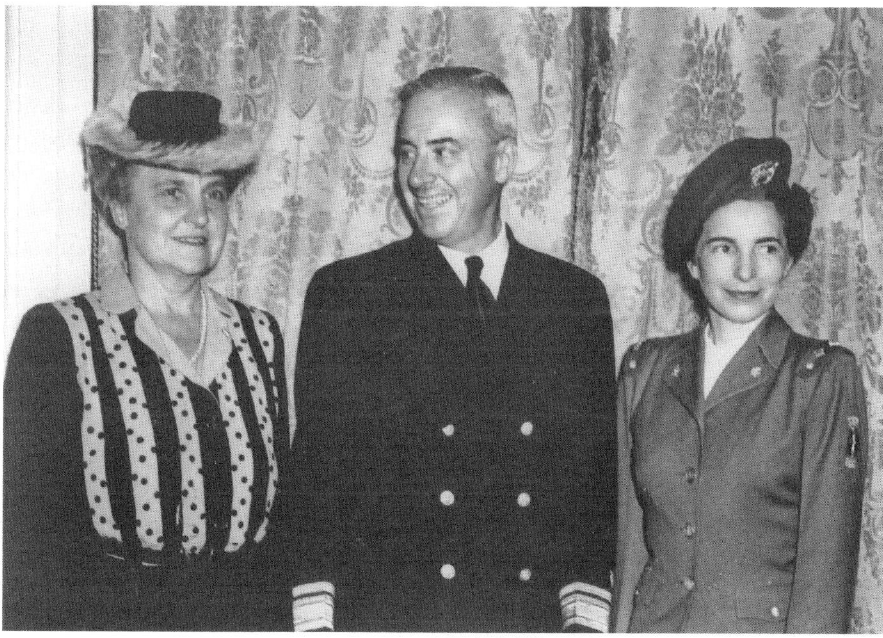

Above: Frances Payne Bolton (left), representative from Ohio and champion of nursing education, introduced legislation in the house on March 29, 1943, that established the Cadet Nurse Corps. Pictured at the right is Lucile Petry, founding director of Nurse Education, U.S. Public Health Service, in her Cadet Nurse Corps uniform. Pictured center is Surgeon General Thomas Parran. *Program Support Center, Department of Health & Human Services.*

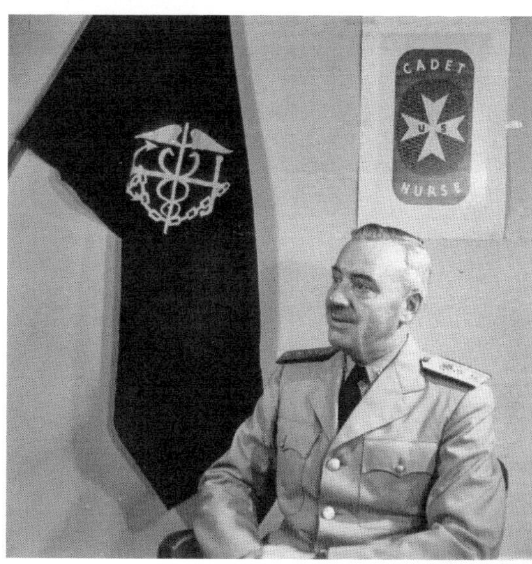

Right: Surgeon General Thomas Parran, U.S. Public Health Service. *U.S. National Library of Medicine.*

Public Health Service, then under the direction of Surgeon General Thomas Parran. Lucile Petry, RN, was the founding director of the Division of Nurse Education, which administered the U.S. Cadet Nurse Corps program. After the war, she became the first chief nurse officer with the rank of assistant surgeon general.

Representative Bolton had introduced HR 2326, Nursing Training Act,[3] earlier in the spring of 1943. Known at that time as the nation's wealthiest woman, Bolton was said to have had a deep regard for nurses because of her extended experiences with nurses who cared for her son, who suffered from a chronic disease. However, her interest in nursing ran much deeper. Bolton was a child of privilege, but as a young woman, she accompanied a visiting nurse on her rounds through the tenements of Cleveland. The young Frances admired their work and resolved to use her fortune and social position to improve the education and professional standing of nurses. She later served on the boards of the Visiting Nurses Association and the Lakeside Hospital Training School in Cleveland and provided funding for the National Organization of Public Health Nurses and for the Case Western Reserve University to set up a school of nursing. She was also instrumental in providing financial support for African American nursing organizations, which, in turn, were the impetus for inclusion of the nondiscrimination clause in the U.S. Cadet Nurse Corps regulations. Congresswoman Bolton saw nursing as the number-one service a constructive professional career for women could perform not only during war but also during peacetime. Bolton arguably saw nurses on the vanguard for social change.[4]

Through the U.S. Cadet Nurse Corps program, the federal government provided qualified schools of nursing funding to cover tuition and fees, stipends and uniforms. Students accepted into the U.S. Cadet Nurse Corps had to be high school graduates between the age of seventeen and thirty-five, be in good health and agree to serve in the nursing profession for the duration of the war to qualify for scholarships, modest stipends and uniforms. Approximately 3,000 African Americans, 350 Japanese and 40 Native Americans became nurses through this program.

The Nurse Training Act of 1943 also provided funding support for curriculum and program development not only for the cadet nurses but also for graduate nurse refresher courses so that experienced nurses who were inactive could return to service in the nation's understaffed hospitals. Expenses associated with needed facility improvements were covered by the already existing Lanham Act of 1940.[5] By making capital improvements, nursing schools in Arizona would be enabled to meet the demand by larger

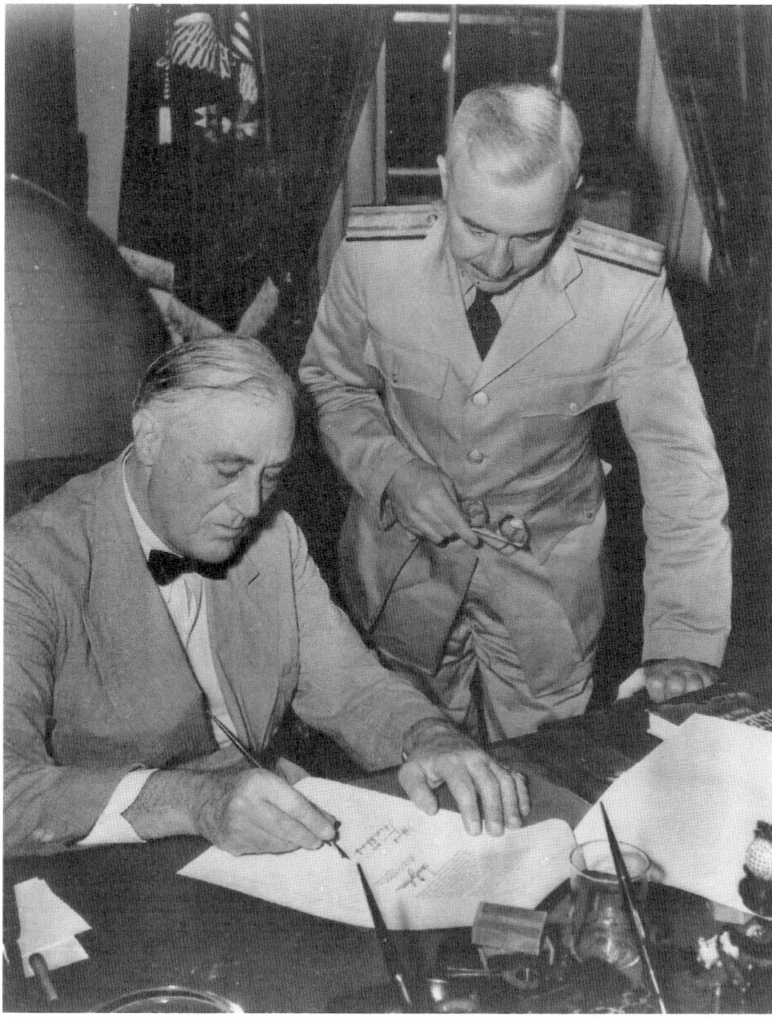

On June 15, 1943, President Roosevelt signed into law the bill that created the Nurse Training Act, which later became known as the Bolton Act. Surgeon General Thomas Parron looks on. *National Archives and Records Administration.*

numbers of student nurses and returning graduate nurses for student housing, libraries and classroom space.

One of the hallmarks of the program was its accelerated thirty-month curriculum with an additional six-month supervised clinical practice as a senior cadet. Through this experience, cadet nurses traveled to other hospitals to learn specialties of interest to them that were not necessarily available in their home hospital. Some Arizona cadet nurses served in Indian Service,

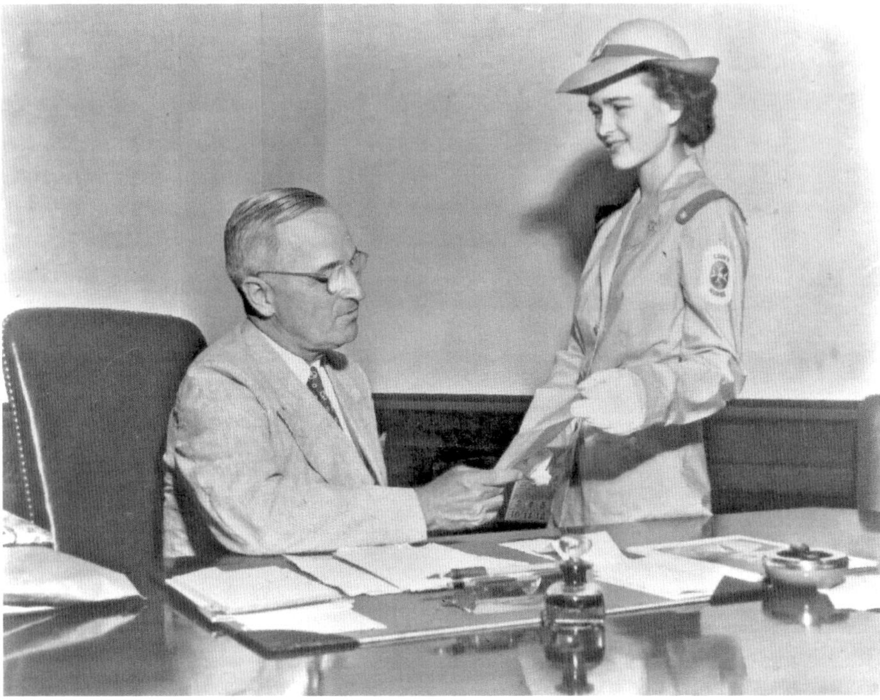

President Harry Truman and Cadet Nurse Helen Hinde reviewed plans for the Cadet Nurse Corps. When the war ended in 1945, cadet nurses in training were allowed to complete their programs of study. The U.S. Cadet Nurse Corps ended in 1948, when the last cadet nurses graduated. *Program Support Center, Department of Health & Human Services (per Thelma Robinson's archive).*

military and veterans hospitals during this period, but the majority remained in their home hospital, where there was also a great need. Not every school of nursing application to participate was accepted into the program. There were specific curricular and facility requirements to be met. A few hundred nursing schools failed to meet the requirements and, in effect, went out of business. None of these schools were located in Arizona.

At the end of the war, the U.S. Cadet Nurse Corps was gradually phased out by President Harry Truman. Cadet nurses already in the pipeline in 1945 at the end of World War II were permitted to complete their program of study. The last cadet nurses graduated, and the program ceased operation in 1948.

Recruitment

According to Beatrice Kalisch and Philip Kalisch,[6] before the Cadet Nurse Corps, nursing received little attention from the general public. Nursing had shied away from publicity, because of the perception that nursing was unprofessional, undesirable, unethical and undignified. Nurses also lacked the ability to present themselves and their cause well. So when the war began and the need to recruit new nurses was apparent, an organizational structure for recruitment was put into place across the country. The War Advertising Council, a collaboration among all the major advertising companies, donated its services to publicity, planning and organizing, persuading others to donate time and space for publicity and getting government backing for its efforts. The services of the then well-known J. Walter Thompson advertising agency were made available to the U.S. Cadet Nurse Corps.

Young women in Arizona might have learned about the U.S. Cadet Nurse Corps because of this well-coordinated campaign, which was run through a partnership of the U.S. Public Health Service and the Office of War Information. Advertisers were advised to emphasize several messaging themes in the local media:

> *A lifetime education without cost—if you can qualify.*
> *Enlist in a proud profession—Become a nurse*
> *The uniform and insignia of the U.S. Cadet Nurse Corps*

For additional information, prospective cadet nurses were directed to their nearest hospital. Advertising material also provided a mailing address to request additional information: U.S. Cadet Nurse Corps, Box 88, New York, NY.

In *How Advertisers Can Cooperate with the U.S. Cadet Nurse Corps*, the guidebook that provided for consistent messaging for Cadet Nurse Corps recruitment efforts, advertisers were advised to direct print material to reach graduates of accredited high schools or colleges through an approach that "will naturally have to be one that appeals to people of character and intelligence."[7] Advertising also had to meet the approval of parents. Parents had to be convinced that "the U.S. Cadet Nurse Corps offers their daughters a rare and valuable opportunity—the opportunity of receiving an education—without cost—of assuring their future with a proud and dependable profession."[8] Nursing was considered war work with a future.

Getting the word out about the U.S. Cadet Nurse Corps in the states was coordinated centrally through the National Nursing Council for War Service, which oversaw the Arizona Nursing Council for War Service. The federal government distributed a manual to facilitate the formation and institutionalization of the Arizona Nursing Council for War Service, as well as a packet of resource materials to assist in the recruitment of student nurses.[9] In these packets were guidance documents on how to approach prospective students in high school or college, elicit inquiries and convert inquiries into enrollment in nursing schools. There were also reprints of pertinent magazine and research articles that could be used with high school or college students and their families. This document outlined the roles and responsibilities of each level of the Nursing Council. There were enrollment goals set for each year that the program operated, and each state was assigned an admissions quota. For example, the national quota for the 1942–43 academic year was 55,000; Arizona's quota for this first year of the program was 170.

Two phases of recruitment were addressed in Arizona: (1) stimulating interest among potential applicants and (2) answering and following up on inquiries so that qualified students were placed appropriately in a school of nursing. Recruitment covered every step necessary to get enough qualified students actually enrolled in approved schools of nursing.

The Arizona State Nursing Council for War Service facilitated relationships among nursing organizations in Arizona, the local media, the State Board of Nursing Examiners and non-nursing groups. These relationships helped these groups collaborate with one another in the coordination of activities designed to increase interest in the program and to ultimately result in enrollment in nursing school. There was a State Committee on Recruitment of Student Nurses, local nursing councils for War Service and local committees on Recruitment of Student Nurses. This effort was viewed as a collaborative one, engaging not only nursing councils but also all possible avenues of communication. "The school has a vital stake in the whole program, as it alone can actually admit and train students."[10]

Prospective cadet nurses in Arizona's high schools might have been approached to apply in response to any number of publicity tools, including ads in magazines, radio broadcasts or newspapers. College students contemplating a career in nursing might have attended a talk at a national convention. Brochures were made available, and recruitment posters were displayed in high schools, colleges, hospitals, store windows and other places where many prospective students would see them. Prospective cadet nurses in Arizona might have seen one of the series of recruitment posters in a theater lobby, a women's shoe store, a beauty shop, a YWCA, a public library or a church. There were Cadet Nurse Corps store window displays in downtown locations and billboard displays along the highways. Prominent local businesses normally donated resources. For example, representative of this type of effort was a full-page, interactive, informative and engaging ad placed in the *Arizona Republic* newspaper during the latter part of the program's operation. At the bottom of the ad was a list of around one hundred businesses, along with the City of Phoenix, all of whom sponsored the ad. Brochures were placed in high schools, physician's offices, schools of nursing and drugstores. Car cards advertising the Cadet Nurse Corps were in streetcars and buses across the country. Arizona's young women might have also heard about the Cadet Nurse Corps through an ad on the radio during soap operas, variety shows, symphony concerts and documentary programs. During the first year of operation, $1.5 million of radio time, representing 700 million listener impressions, was donated to the corps.

Cadet nurses were also highlighted in dramatizations and were on occasion written into a story line in the entertainment media. Prospective Arizona cadet nurses might have seen newsreels about the program in the movie houses. One clip showed President Roosevelt signing the Bolton Act and another featured the modeling of the new cadet corps' uniforms.

Many moviegoers in the 1940s were teenagers, which prompted the release of *Reward Unlimited*. This Selznick production featured Dorothy McGuire in the starring role as Peggy Adams, a young woman who wanted to serve her country, learned about the U.S. Cadet Nurse Corps and joined the program. It was arguably the best recruitment film in 1944 and was presented at sixteen thousand movie theaters with an estimated audience of ninety million. Later during the war years, 16mm prints were made available to community organization, such as YWCAs, parent-teacher associations, church groups, civic clubs and high school and college assemblies.

Young women and their parents in Arizona might have heard the radio play *This Is Our War*, which is about Sally Kimball, who eventually recognized her responsibilities to her nation and joined the Cadet Nurse Corps. This short play was received well and thought to be among the best special purpose plays written during the war.

The Arizona State Nursing Council was tasked with the responsibility to maintain contact with every high school, preparatory school, junior college and particularly every college within the state to make sure that each had recruitment posters, vocational literature and speakers on recruitment who

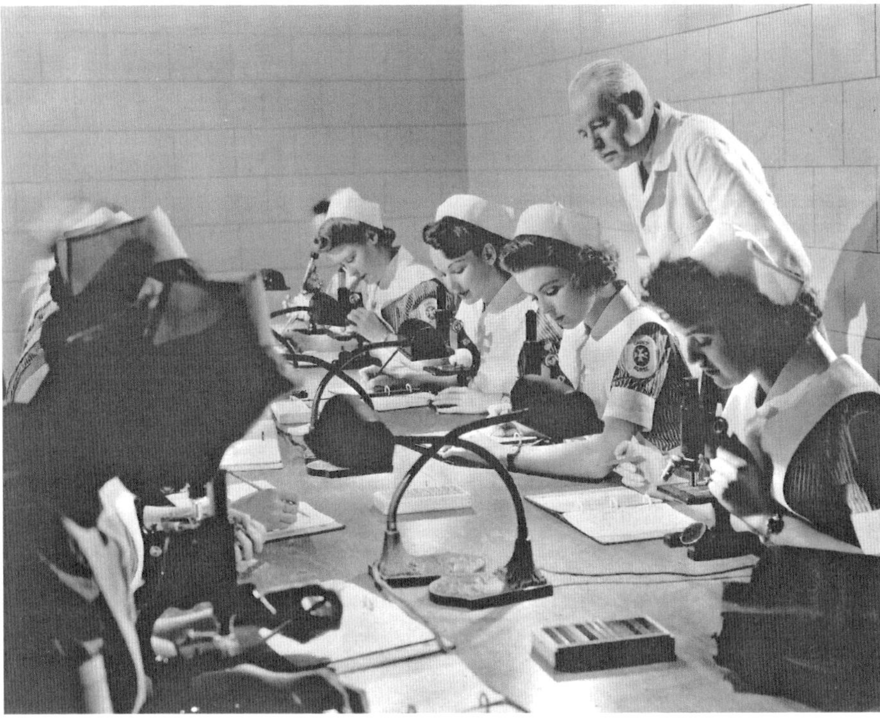

Actress Dorothy McGuire, in character as Peggy Adams, is pictured here among fellow cadet nurses receiving instruction in the bacteriology laboratory in the film *Reward Unlimited*, the U.S. Cadet Nurse Corps short-subject feature produced for the U.S. Public Health Service. *Author's collection.*

could consult with students, counselors and parents. This responsibility also included providing opportunities for interested students to visit a school of nursing and get firsthand impressions.

Representative of this multi-prong recruitment effort was a Cadet Nurse Corps interview simulation that took place in Tucson High School. The *Kingman Mohave Miner* reported that prospective students were interviewed by Cadet Nurses at Saint Mary's Hospital School of Nursing who were assigned as special nurse recruiters during National Cadet Nurse Recruitment Week in April 1945. The same paper ran recruitment ads, based on a centrally developed template, to attract female high school students to consider nursing as a lifetime career.

Over one hundred local Phoenix-area businesses took out a full page Cadet Nurse Corps recruitment ad in the *Arizona Republic* newspaper. Its message was brought by "patriotic firms and individuals in the interest of the nation's urgent war activities." In this ad, Cadet Nurse activities and opportunities were described, and readers were offered a self-test that contained these questions:

> *Are you between 17 and 35 years of age?*
> *Are you in good health?*
> *Have you graduated from an accredited high school or have you had some college education?*
> *Are you interested in science?*
> *Have you a sense of humor?*
> *Have you an orderly mind?*
> *Are you deft with your hands?*
> *Are you neat?*
> *Are you quick to grasp what you see, read and hear?*
> *Are you interested in people?*

There was also a reply form that could be filled out and sent to New York for more information for schools of nursing outside Arizona, or the reader could phone Mrs. Ida Colburn locally.

Of all of the recruitment efforts during World War II, the U.S. Cadet Nurse Corps was most successful; it met all of its recruitment targets. An estimated 180,000 women nationally volunteered to serve through this program. Of that number, about 124,000 completed nurse training and became registered nurses. Their average length of service in nursing of at least twenty-eight years went far beyond their promise to serve for the duration of the war. There were some 1,125 participating schools of nurses nationally, including 7 in Puerto Rico. Pennsylvania, New York, Illinois and Ohio had the largest numbers of participating schools of nursing, representing about 32 percent of all participating schools of nursing nationally. According to Furman & Williams:

> *Of all students entering schools of nursing approved by State boards of nurse examiners, 70 percent in 1943, 88.5 percent in 1944, and 70 percent in 1945 were members of the U.S. Cadet Nurse Corps.*
>
> *At the height of the program, Senior Cadets supplied 80 percent of the nursing service in the institutions which operated the nursing schools participating in the program. About half of the 35,000 Senior Cadets who applied for Federal service in the last year of the war were assigned to the Veterans Administration, the rest going into Army, Indian Service, and Public Health Service hospitals.*[11]

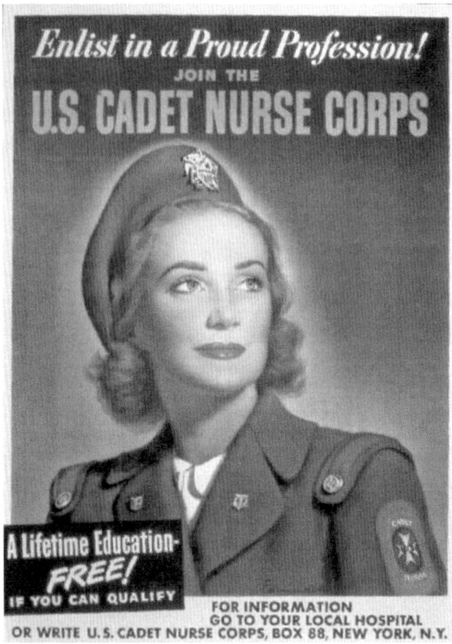

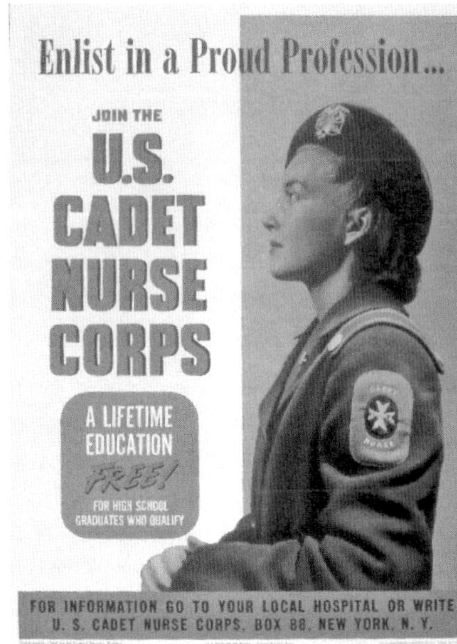

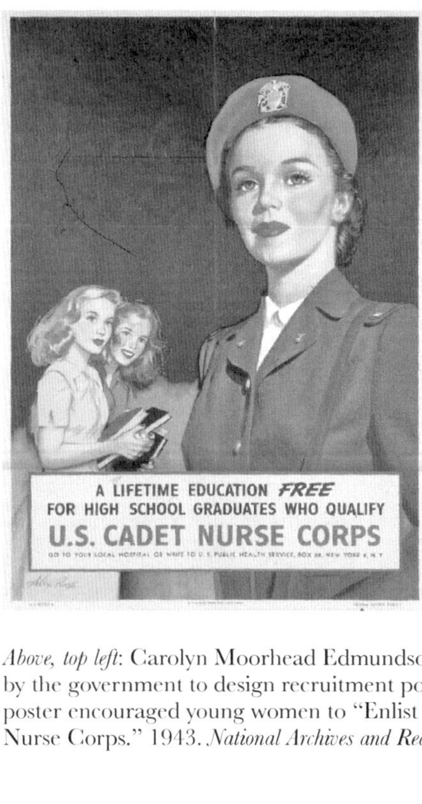

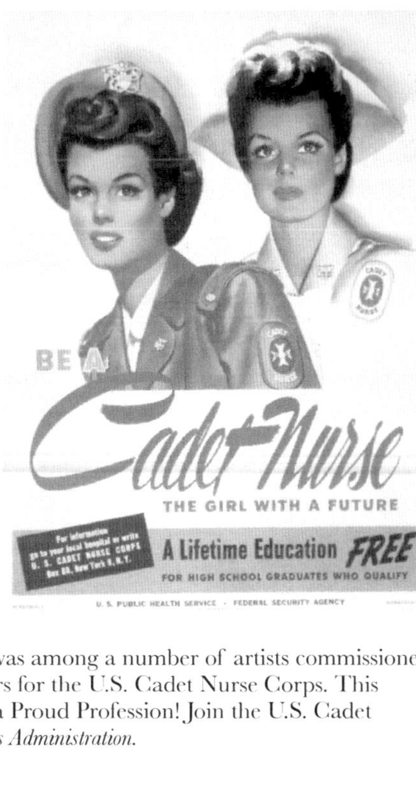

Above, top left: Carolyn Moorhead Edmundson was among a number of artists commissioned by the government to design recruitment posters for the U.S. Cadet Nurse Corps. This poster encouraged young women to "Enlist in a Proud Profession! Join the U.S. Cadet Nurse Corps." 1943. *National Archives and Records Administration.*

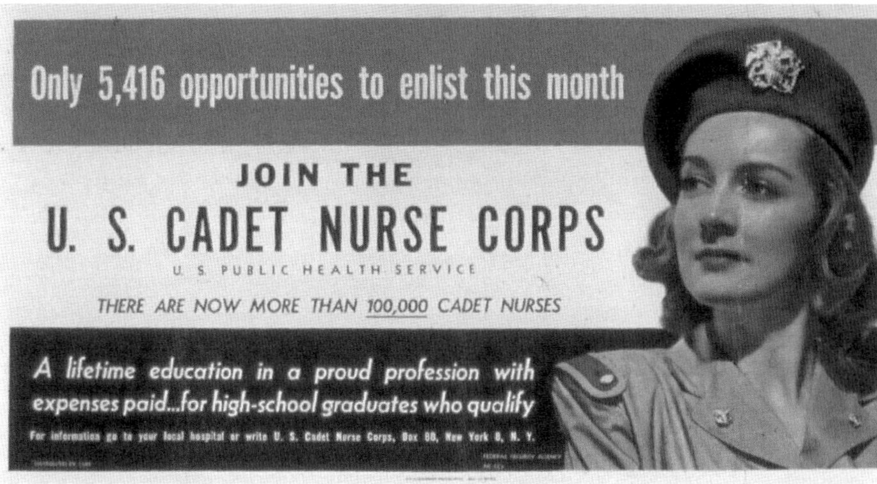
Only 5,416 opportunities to enlist this month
JOIN THE
U. S. CADET NURSE CORPS
U. S. PUBLIC HEALTH SERVICE
THERE ARE NOW MORE THAN 100,000 CADET NURSES
A lifetime education in a proud profession with expenses paid...for high-school graduates who qualify
For information go to your local hospital or write U. S. Cadet Nurse Corps, Box 88, New York 8, N. Y.

Above: Through this poster, young women were invited to "join the U.S. Cadet Nurse Corps." *National Archives and Records Administration.*

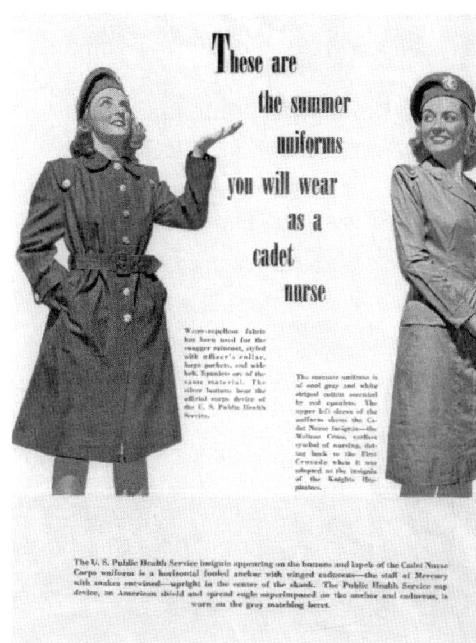
These are the summer uniforms you will wear as a cadet nurse
The U. S. Public Health Service insignia appearing on the buttons and lapels of the Cadet Nurse Corps uniform is a horizontal fouled anchor with winged caduceus—the staff of Mercury with snakes entwined—upright in the center of the shank. The Public Health Service cap device, an American shield and spread eagle superimposed on the anchor and caduceus, is worn on the gray matching beret.

Right: Young women in Arizona may have seen this display showing them what the summer Cadet Nurse Corps uniforms looked like. The summer uniform is of cool gray and white striped cotton accented by red epaulets. The upper left sleeve of the uniform shows the cadet nurse insignia—the Maltese Cross, earliest symbol of nursing, dating back to the First Crusade when it was adopted as the insignia of the Knights Hospitalers. *National Archives and Records Administration.*

Opposite, top right: This poster encouraged young women and their parents to obtain information about the U.S. Cadet Nurse Corps by going to a local hospital or writing to U.S. Cadet Nurse Corps, Box 88, New York, N.Y. 1942. *National Archives and Records Administration.*

Opposite, bottom left: Alexander Ross was another artist commissioned by the government to design a recruitment poster for the U.S. Cadet Nurse Corps. This poster reminded young women that the program offered "a lifetime education FREE for high school graduates who qualify." 1945. *University of North Texas Digital Library*

Opposite, bottom right: Jon Whitcomb was a third artist commissioned by the government to design a recruitment poster for the U.S. Cadet Nurse Corps. This poster invited young women to "be a cadet nurse—The girl with a future." *National Archives and Records Administration.*

The total cost to the government of the five-year U.S. Cadet Nurse Corps program was $149,026,478, roughly equivalent to some $1,473,830,000 in 2014. The per student cost of training to the federal government averaged $1,360, or approximately $13,450 in 2014. This amount did not cover the full cost of educating and training nurses, but it did cover all costs that would have normally been charged to the student over the course of the full three-year program.[12] Recruitment costs were $92 per student (around $1,218 in 2014), of which $82 (about $1,085 in 2014) came in the form of in-kind contributions.[13]

Chapter 2

ARIZONA DURING WORLD WAR II

In order to provide a better understanding of the U.S. Cadet Nurse Corps in Arizona, in this chapter I offer a brief overview of World War II Arizona. This overview will set the context in which cadet nurses in Arizona were situated—a time before interstate highways and air conditioning in the still Wild West. This overview is important, lest we forget that the Arizona of the 1940s was different from what it has become in the twenty-first century. We can conclude that how a place feels in the present day has roots in history, and this overview may be helpful in tracing the historical context and roots for some of today's generally accepted assumptions about nursing education and practice. It is through this overview that I hope to clarify Cadet Nurse Corps' aims and purpose.

Arizona became a state in 1912, so at less than thirty years old when World War II began, Arizona was relatively young. However, as a region, this formerly northern frontier of Mexico had a much longer history tracing back to pre-Columbian times. Mexican culture and Spanish language, as well as the indigenous cultures with a longer history, were an indelible part of the landscape for many decades before Arizona statehood. Arizona had a rich, long history that included the movement of peoples and goods headed for other parts of North, Central and South America. Arizona, along with much of the U.S. Southwest, also received many Native American peoples who were pushed westward by eastern settlers. Among these peoples in Arizona were the Navajo, Hopi and Apache tribes. The Navajo Code Talkers were instrumental in the defeat of the Japanese during World War

II, though no one in Arizona would have known of their work during the war. The code talkers were sworn to secrecy until 1964. This multicultural heritage, which was developed over centuries, continues to be felt to this day in Arizona. Others have written detailed accounts of this history,[14] so we will not dwell on this foundational history here. Neither will we dwell on the sometimes tense relationship between the United States and Mexico because of a history of broken promises made with Mexican contract workers and employers in the western states' agricultural industry.[15]

At the beginning of World War II, the United States maintained a neutral posture and did not engage in the war effort. After the bombing of Pearl Harbor and with increased pressure from our British allies, who were suffering terribly in their attempts to keep the Axis from entering Great Britain, everything changed. The United States began to produce all sorts of equipment—ammunition, transports, tanks and aircraft equipped with magnetron No. 12 radar—in an effort to equip not only an inexperienced American military but also British allies to defeat the Axis powers. The United States entered an industrial and social revolution that was especially felt in the West. It was as if, as David Kennedy put it,[16] the North American continent was tipped, and everything—people, money and machinery—just slid westward across the country. During this time the population of California grew 53 percent, Oregon by 40 percent and Washington State by 37 percent. Women became the core of the labor force. Across the country, around nineteen million women worked in war factories, the transportation industry and agriculture. This period was not called a production miracle for no reason. Cadet nurses in Arizona were training at a time when there was a lot of other war work going on around them, and there were many occupational choices for women that had not existed previously.

Topographically, Arizona had been a sparsely populated state with a harsh desert climate in the southern part, and the northern part was home to ponderosa pines and some of the nation's most majestic beauty, such as the Grand Canyon and the Colorado River. Over 40 percent of Arizona's landmass was and continues to be federally owned. These public lands included national parks, forests, wildlife refuges, monuments, wilderness areas and lands managed by the Bureau of Land Management. Approximately 25 percent of the state's territory was sovereign land of Native American nations, including Navajo, Hopi, Yaqui and Colorado River tribes, courtesy of federal policy and administrative oversight by the Bureau of Indian Affairs. With so much federally owned and sovereign land, Arizona was vulnerable to pressure to host a number of war-related facilities. For example, the federal government authorized the building of Japanese internment camps in Arizona on Native American reservation land over the objection of Native American communities. However, the predominant message in the media was that supporting the war effort—by buying war bonds or by working in the defense industry, for example—was a patriotic act.

During World War II, Arizona was home to twenty-four prisoner-of-war camps, five of which were base camps. There was a base prisoner-of-war camp in five of Arizona's then fourteen counties, and two base camps in Yuma County. The state was also home to two military training facilities and a recreational area for military officers returning from the battlefield and needing R&R.

Cadet nurses in Phoenix trained within miles of a number of these POW camps and undoubtedly heard about the escape of German POWs from the Papago Camp in Phoenix on December 23, 1944. One of the escapees had traveled to within ten miles of the Mexican border, and all either turned themselves in or were captured by the end of January 1945. Cadet nurses in Phoenix and Tucson were also within about fifty miles of the nation's largest all-new prisoner of war compound, the first ever constructed on American soil, Camp Florence, where there were 5,500 German POW detainees. Arizona POW camps imprisoned over 13,000 of the 370,000 German POWs and more than 600 of the 51,000 Italian Service Unit POWs detained in the United States during World War II.[17]

There was a forty-fold increase in the size of the U.S. military with some sixteen million soldiers nationally—13 percent of the U.S. population. Cadet nurses in Arizona were not too far away from a number of record-breaking military facilities. One was the Desert Training Center, also known as the California-Arizona Maneuver Area (DTC/CAMA). The DTC/CAMA was activated on April 1, 1942. It was a training facility to prepare U.S. Army and army air corps units and personnel to live and fight in the desert, to test and develop equipment and to develop tactical techniques and training methods. It was a key training facility for units engaged in combat during the 1942–43 North African campaign. The DTC/CAMA stretched from Southern California to within 50 miles west of Phoenix and in Arizona from Yuma in the south to the southern tip of Nevada at the north. It was approximately 350 miles wide and 250 miles long. These training grounds directly impacted more than one million troops.

This simulated theater of operation was the largest military training ground in the history of military maneuvers and included the DTC headquarters, the world's largest army post, which was headquartered in

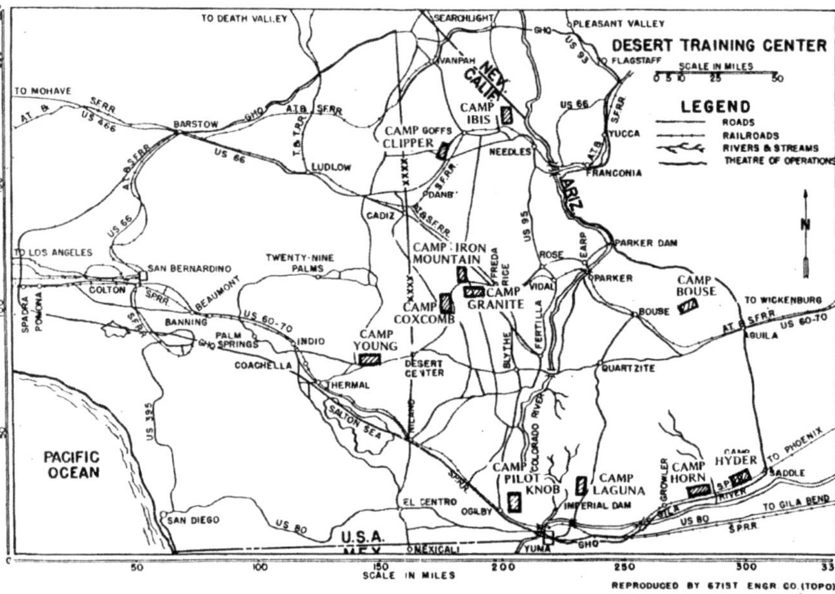

Desert Training Center map. *U.S. Army via United States Bureau of Land Management.*

California. Major General George S. Patton Jr. was the first commanding general of the DTC. Over time, the DTC expanded its scope from a training ground for combat in North Africa to a theater of operations to train combat troops, service units and staffs for service anywhere overseas. It closed on July 1, 1944, a year after the beginning of the U.S. Cadet Nurse Corps program.

During World War II, many military wives and girlfriends followed their husbands or boyfriends to their stateside military posts across the country. Such was the case at Fort Huachuca, in southeastern Arizona, about one hundred miles southeast of Tucson, Fort Huachuca housed the nation's largest contingent of African American soldiers in the then segregated U.S. Army. African American army wives lived in a harsh setting, a setting that would be in stark contrast to that of cadet nurses' living arrangements elsewhere in the state. According to Thelma Thurston Gorham's 1943 account, "Negro Army Wives," African American army wives "closed their eyes and ears to the fact that white civilian workers were furnished far more livable lodgings."

Cadet nurses in Phoenix were literally within miles of other military training facilities. One was a collaboration between a private American flight school and the British Royal Air Force, called the British Flying Training

School No. 4. It was located at Falcon Field in Mesa. This training facility was one of six in the United States; the other five were scattered across four other states: Florida, Texas, California and Oklahoma. Falcon Field was a five-hundred-acre facility. Originally to be named Thunderbird Air Field No. 3, Falcon Field came from the British aviators themselves, according to many, who wanted a familiar predatory bird to them as a symbol for their training and abilities. The first cadets arrived in 1941 and trained in good weather and wide-open terrain. A lack of enemy airpower provided safer and more efficient training than was possible in England. Nonetheless, twenty-three British cadets, one American cadet and four instructors were killed and are now buried in Mesa City Cemetery. Several thousand pilots were trained there until the RAF installation was closed at the end of the war. In addition to Falcon Field, Southwest Airways operated three other flight training schools in what is now metropolitan Phoenix. The Thunderbird School of Global Management occupies what was once Thunderbird No. 1 airfield. Scottsdale Airpark was originally Thunderbird No. 2, and Southwest Airways' first airfield grew into what is now known as Sky Harbor Airport.

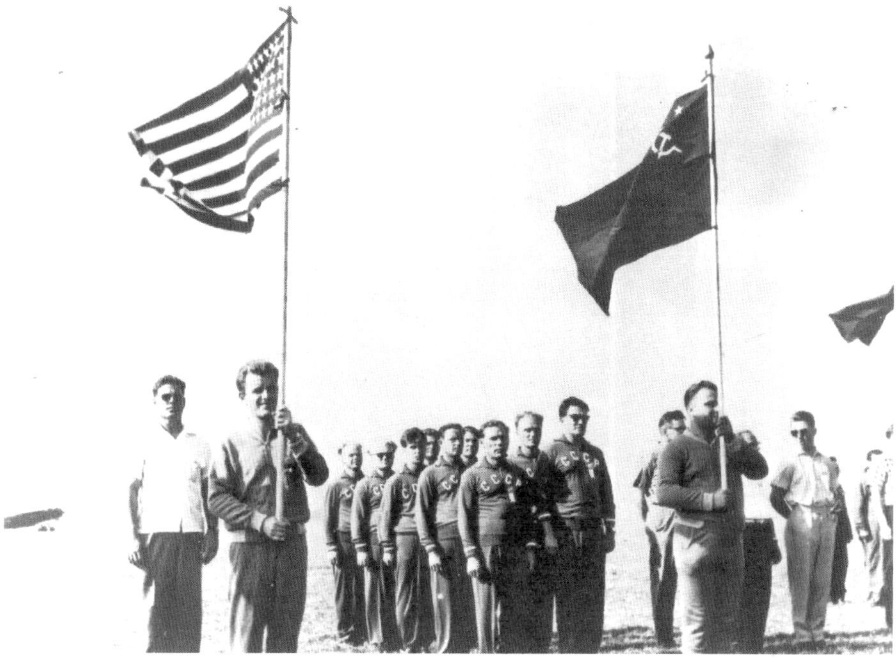

American and Soviet color guards side by side at Falcon Field during World War II. Date unknown. *Falcon Field Airport, City of Mesa.*

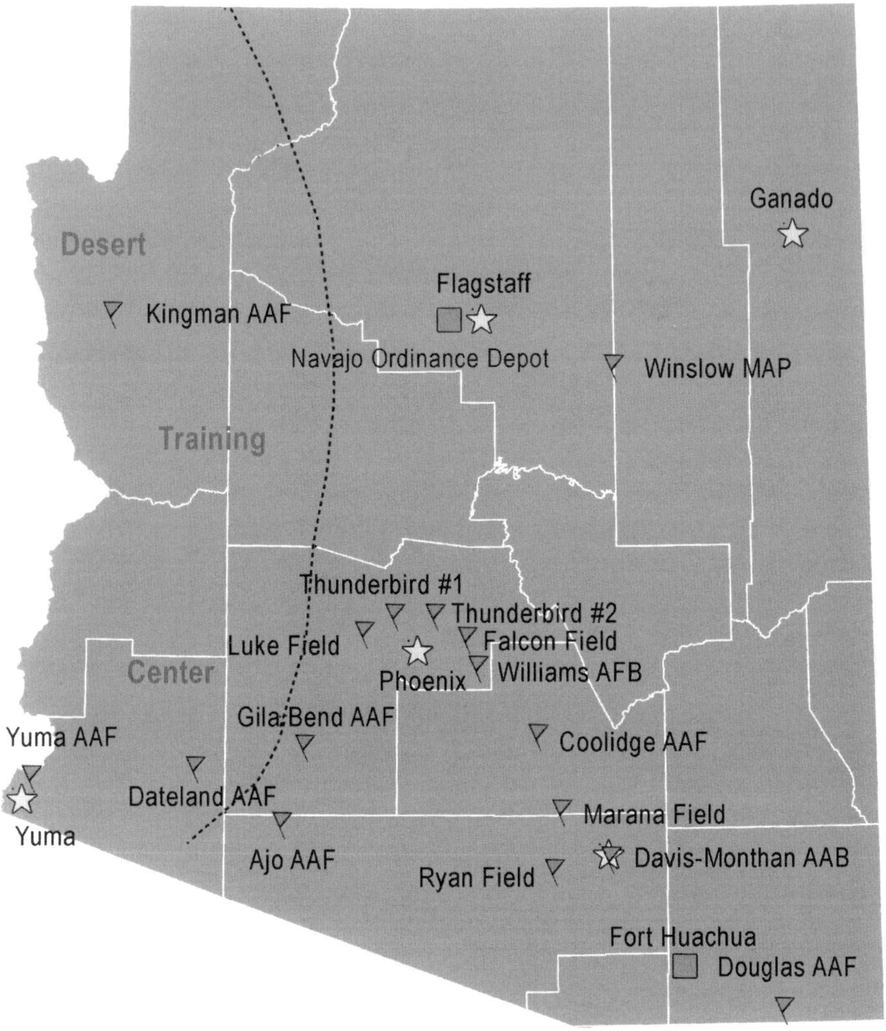

Military installations in Arizona during World War II. *Illustration by author.*

These privately operated flight schools trained pilots for the army air force, as well as cadets from other allied countries.

Nisei—Americans of Japanese ancestry—in nursing schools in western states during the early 1940s after the bombing of Pearl Harbor, experienced interruptions in their training, as they were evacuated to assembly centers for placement in relocation camps. Nisei student nurses in Arizona schools of nursing faced this challenge; if the school of nursing was located in what was known as a "military zone," there was no sanctuary to be found, even in the school itself. One example of this is Mabel Ujiie's story.

Because she was of Japanese heritage and because Good Samaritan Hospital was in the "military zone" in Phoenix, Arizona, Mabel Ujiie was evacuated to Camp Mayer in Mayer, Arizona, in the spring of 1942 and was not permitted to stay in her program of study at Good Samaritan. She was within six months of finishing her training. Ujiie eventually lived in the Poston Relocation Camp in western Arizona, near Parker. (This camp will be discussed later in greater detail.)

From May 6, 1942, to May 5, 1943, numerous attempts were made to arrange for the continuation of Ujiie's training to its completion. These attempts were reflected in correspondence among a number of officials at Good Samaritan Hospital School of Nursing, the War Relocation Council, other federal agencies and officials at other schools of nursing.

At Camp Mayer, Ujiie reported being the only person in the camp with nurse's training and that she was unofficially helping a physician there. On May 8, 1942, Fannie Furth, director of nurses at Good Samaritan, requested that Ujiie be permitted to return to Good Samaritan to finish her studies. The response from Dr. Harrison at the U.S. Public Health Service Office in San Francisco was that a nurse would be assigned to Camp Mayer and that Ujiie would be very helpful as an assistant. He would ask the Assembly Center manager to give her official status in the infirmary. However, this experience would not carry credit toward her program of study because of state regulations.

Ujiie's problem was not uncommon in the western states. Nursing school officials in this region worked to find alternative placements for students of Japanese ancestry so that they could complete their studies in a midwestern or eastern nursing school, where Japanese Americans were not evacuated and interned. The coordinating mechanism for this effort was the National Student Relocation Council. The council was formed at the request of the War Relocation Authority to aid in the relocation of students who were evacuated from the West Coast war zones and wished to continue their studies on the college or university level. In early 1943, Ujiie applied to the National Student Relocation Council for assistance in obtaining an alternative placement to complete her nurse's training.

In the meantime, James Chamberlain Baker, resident bishop of the California Area of the Methodist Church, was in touch with Mrs. J.O. Sexson, RN, superintendent of Good Samaritan Hospital, inquiring as to Ujiie's religious affiliation. He, too, was attempting to find a placement for her, and this information could be helpful. Sexson contacted Dr. Clarence

Salsbury, director of Sage Memorial Hospital in Ganado, Arizona, about the possibilities of placing Ujiie at Sage to continue her studies there, as Ganado was apparently outside the "military zone."

By the end of January 1943, Woodruff J. Emlen of the Placement Department at the National Student Relocation Council, West Coast Committee, in San Francisco, wanted to know if Good Samaritan Hospital was located in the military district. If so, then Ujiie would not be permitted to return to Good Samaritan to complete her studies.

At the beginning of February 1943, Vivian R. Biggar, the next director of nurses at Good Samaritan Hospital, inquired of Pauline Brown at the Office of War Information about whether Nisei girls could continue nursing school elsewhere in the United States. This option was already available to Nisei boys who wished to serve in the military or to finish college. If so, she would like to reinstate Ujiie. Biggar sought the support of the Office of War Information in this case.

By February 1943, Ujiie was living at the Poston Relocation Camp in western Arizona when she received a letter from Biggar, the director of Good Samaritan's school of nursing, summarizing various parties' efforts to have her return to Good Samaritan to finish there or to transfer to Sage Memorial Hospital and complete her studies there. The latter option appeared to be the better one, and Biggar advised Ujiie to contact Dr. Salsbury as soon as possible.

Through her application with the National Student Relocation Council, administrators at a Chicago school of nursing were considering admitting Ujiie into their program. In a response to a request for a letter of recommendation, on March 12, 1943, Biggar reported to the director of Walther Memorial Hospital in Chicago, Illinois, that the City of Phoenix had been put "In Bounds" and that Ujiie would be able to return to Good Samaritan to complete her course of study. Ujiie did return to Good Samaritan and finished in 1943. She was not permitted to count any of the clinical experiences that she encountered in Mayer or in Poston. Mabel Ujiie's entry into the nursing profession was delayed a full year.

Although Mabel Ujiie's situation predated the U.S. Cadet Nurse Corps by a year, her story illustrates some of the tensions of wartime Arizona in which cadet nurses found themselves during their training years. Officials did communicate with one another between the schools of nursing and tried to help one another solve difficult problems. That there were so many military installations, prisoner-of-war detention facilities and relocation camps housing Americans of Japanese heritage so close to one another in this state did affect hospital schools of nursing. Not only did many nurses leave the hospitals to help in the war effort as military nurses, but it was also difficult to find replacements for them because older graduate nurses had left employment for other personal reasons, such as marriage and raising children. Even when they did, there was no guarantee that all nurses in training would be able to complete their training without interruption.

Mabel Ujiie was not the only young woman whose training was interrupted and dreams delayed. A number of young women in the state's two relocation camps were similarly affected. Arizona was home to seven relocation facilities to address what was known as the Japanese problem in the western states. During what some might call one of the darkest periods of U.S. history, Nisei were removed from their homes and detained in a number of internment camps located in the western United States. In Arizona, there were two relocation camps, an assembly center, a reception center and three isolation or detention centers. The relocation camps—Gila River south of Phoenix and Poston in the middle of the Desert Training Center—were located on Indian Reservation land in Arizona. The assembly center in Mayer operated for a very short time during 1942 to receive persons of Japanese descent from southern Arizona into the Poston facility. At their peaks, the Poston and Gila River Relocation Centers housed 17,814 people and 13,348 people, respectively, making these two facilities the third- and fourth-largest cities in Arizona after Phoenix and Tucson. These two facilities were also the second and third largest of the ten relocation centers, housing approximately 30 percent of the 104,106 Americans of Japanese origin unfortunate enough to be living in the western United States during World War II.

According to *Confinement and Ethnicity*, the relocation centers were designed to be self-contained communities. In addition to housing, there were hospitals, post offices, schools, warehouses, offices and factories. However, patients with more serious illnesses or injuries would be transferred to a better-equipped hospital, such as Saint Joseph's Hospital in Phoenix.

Each camp had a main entrance leading to the local highway and auxiliary routes to farming areas outside the central core. Some of the major interior roads were paved, but most were simply dirt roads that were dusty or muddy depending on the weather. Most of the camps were surrounded by barbed wire and guard towers. However, since Gila River and Poston were located on dead-end streets, they were less guarded.

Since the centers were supposed to be as self-sufficient as possible, the residential core was surrounded by a large buffer zone that also served as farmland. Military and civilian employees lived separately from the residents to reduce fraternization. Living quarters were available to civilian employees at the camp but were generally supplemented by available housing in nearby towns.

A number of young women in Gila River became cadet nurses, thereby affording them the opportunity to leave the camp. Alice Coguchi Kanagaki and her family were ordered to leave their Vacaville, California, home in April 1942 and arrived in Gila River some five months later,[18] after a period of time in the Turlock Assembly Center in California. By her account, there were hospitals staffed by physicians, registered nurses and auxiliary help, though limited equipment and skilled personnel also limited health outcomes for patients. Schools were established, credentialed and staffed by qualified teachers from within the camp or who were volunteers from outside. Though the high school curriculum was limited, it was adequate for college preparation.

Alice remembered:

> *As a teenager in the junior and senior years, I did not realize the dedication and sacrifice involved in these Caucasian teachers who volunteered to come to these desolate areas to teach a group of students, a group of people whom they knew so little about, as few Japanese people lived in Arizona or other states where the relocation camps were built.*
>
> *These volunteer teachers were surprised to find that the Japanese American students were bright and eager to learn and presented very few disciplinary problems. These teachers in turn provided the encouragement and support for the students to perform to the best of their abilities and to continue on to higher education. The percentage of students going on to college from these camps was higher than the national average.*

Alice was inspired by a registered nurse who worked in the camp hospital. During Alice's senior year in high school, a cousin in Wisconsin wrote and told her about the U.S. Cadet Nurse Corps. She suggested that Alice apply. Alice did and was accepted into the program in a school of nursing in Madison, Wisconsin. Her three brothers all served in the military during World War II.

Alice added:

> *I was proud of the fact that my brothers were in the service as the general attitude was to prove to all that we were indeed loyal and worthy citizens, and why not? After all, we were born in the United States; we were citizens and knew no other country or culture.*

Ida Sakohira Kawaguchi was another young woman at Gila River who went into the U.S. Cadet Nurse Corps.[19] She was in the last high school graduating class in her hometown of Fowler, California, where her father owned his own grape ranch. Shortly after her high school graduation, she and her family moved to Gila River. While there, she enrolled in nurse aide classes that were offered at the camp hospital. Ida admired and looked up to the Japanese American registered nurses.

After a year of internment, Ida heard about the U.S. Cadet Nurse Corps. She filled out an application form to clear her leave from the internment camp and applied to several schools of nursing. She was accepted at the Saint Mary's School of Nursing in Rochester, Minnesota. Ida reported that the day she left camp was a sad one for her. It was the first time she would be away from her family for such a long period of time. She was scared, as this was the first time she would be on her own.

Grace Obata Amemiya completed two years of pre-nursing studies in California before internment, first at Turlock Assembly Center in California and ultimately at Gila River Relocation Center in Arizona.[20] In Gila River, she worked as a nurse aide in the camp hospital for more than a year and began searching for a school of nursing that would be willing to admit her. During World War II, many schools of nursing were reluctant to admit Japanese Americans out of fear that professional staff or patients would not be able to trust them. She was ultimately accepted into the Saint Mary's Hospital School of Nursing in Rochester, Minnesota, which also made her eligible to join the U.S. Cadet Nurse Corps. She was one of more than seven thousand senior cadet nurses who served in a military hospital as part of her training.

The Catalina Federal Honor Camp was a minimum-security prison labor camp that held men of Japanese descent who were draft resisters or conscientious objectors. It was originally built through an agreement among the Bureau of Prisons, the Bureau of Public Roads and the Arizona Highway Commission. Gordeon Hirabayashi, who had challenged the exclusion of Japanese Americans from the West Coast, was the first Japanese laborer held here. Conscientious objectors who had resisted the draft (e.g., Jehovah's Witnesses, Hopi, Pentecostals and Mennonites) were held here. Inmates at the camp performed road work for what would become the Catalina Highway near Tucson. They drilled holes for dynamite, broke rocks with sledgehammers and cleared trees, as well as grew food and cooked for the prison population. These draft resisters were later pardoned, but the prison remained open until the highway was completed in 1951, when the camp became a labor camp for juvenile offenders.

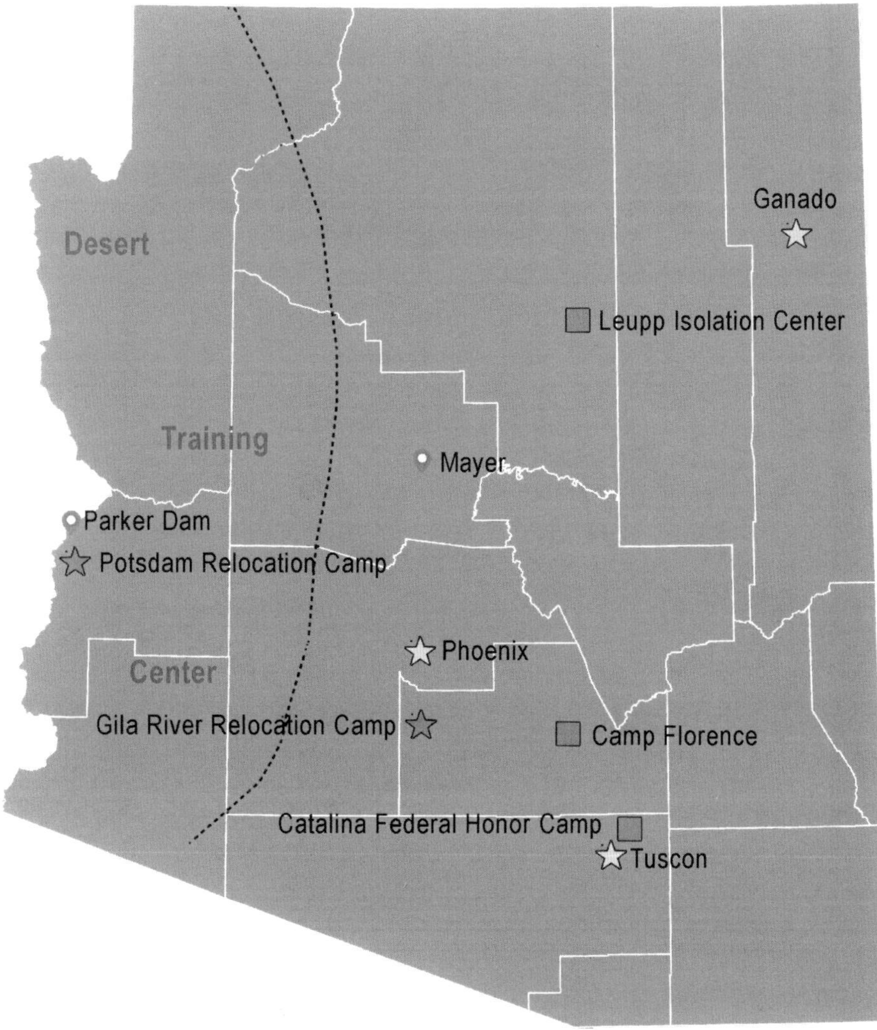

Detention centers in Arizona during World War II. *Illustration by author.*

Another facility for resisters was the Leupp Isolation Center, located on Navajo Nation Reservation lands. The facility was an abandoned Indian Boarding School that was under the authority of the Bureau of Indian Affairs. It operated for less than a year, during 1943, and housed "non-compliant" Japanese "troublemakers." Among the most notorious prisoners at Leupp was Harry Ueno, who led the Manzanar Riot. According to Harry Ueno, the Leupp Isolation Center served similar purposes for Japanese during 1943 as previously with Indian children:

> [They] *used to put the Indian children in the jail under the administration office...It seems that those "cellars" were used to hold Japanese American men and Indian children alike. Young people who had been torn from their families might have been punished for speaking their non-English, traditional language, and like the Japanese American prisoners of relocation camps, the students in the boarding school could be punished for infractions at the discretion of the school commissioner.*

Arizona's population during and after World War II was a story of growth and expansion. In 1940, the population of Arizona was less than 500,000; by 1950, it had grown to 750,000. The population of Phoenix in 1940 was 65,000, but it swelled when the GIs returned home. By 1960, Phoenix had become the largest city in the Southwest with a population of 439,000.[21] All of these people would need healthcare, and cadet nurses in training during the war would be prepared to serve the built-up demand that would unfold with the beginning of the postwar baby boom.

The Arizona that cadet nurses lived in during World War II was a kaleidoscope of compartmentalized war-related activity overlaid on an already historically contested region of the United States. Native Americans were contained on reservations, and Mexicans were segregated from Anglos in the mining industry, for examples. The U.S. Cadet Nurse Corps started operation the same year as Mexican Americans were beginning to press for their civil rights. With World War II came the outright oppression of additional ethnic groups—Germans, Italians and Japanese. All of these groups were confined either through formal government policy or by social circumstance, and among the members of each of these groups were some who pointed out the inequities of the time.

Simultaneously, all of these differences appeared to be subsumed into a larger mission that bound all Arizonans, regardless of race, ethnicity or gender, to put aside these differences and address a threat to all Americans during World War II, especially after the bombing of Pearl Harbor. During this time, the American people were encouraged to pull together toward a greater good. They purchased war bonds to pay for the financial cost of the war, and they opened their homes to war workers and others committed to defeating the enemy. This patriotic fervor undoubtedly permeated everyone across racial, ethnic and other categories. The U.S. Cadet Nurse Corps offered young women in Arizona an opportunity to participate patriotically through service in the state's understaffed hospitals. The program also promised lifelong benefits in this profession with a future.

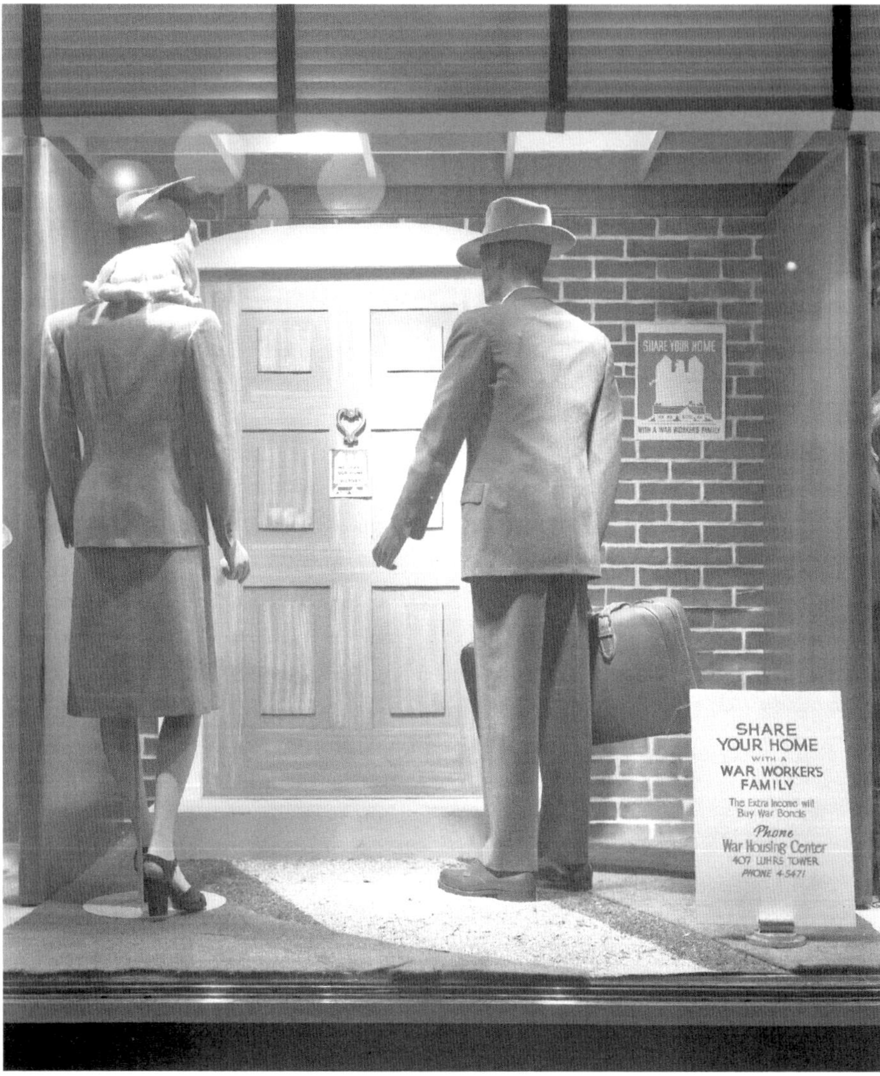

A War Housing Center window display. A sign at Vic Hanny's men's clothing store reads, "Share your Home with a War Worker's Family / The Extra Income will Buy War Bonds / Phone / War Housing Center / 407 Luhrs Tower / PHONE 4-5471." *McCulloch Brothers Inc. Photographs, CP MCLMB. Arizona State University Libraries: Arizona Collection.*

Arizona was one of only a few states in the country, if not the only state of the country, with such a cultural mix. It had always been a north–south trade route for the exchange of goods and people to and from Latin America to the South and the rest of the western North American

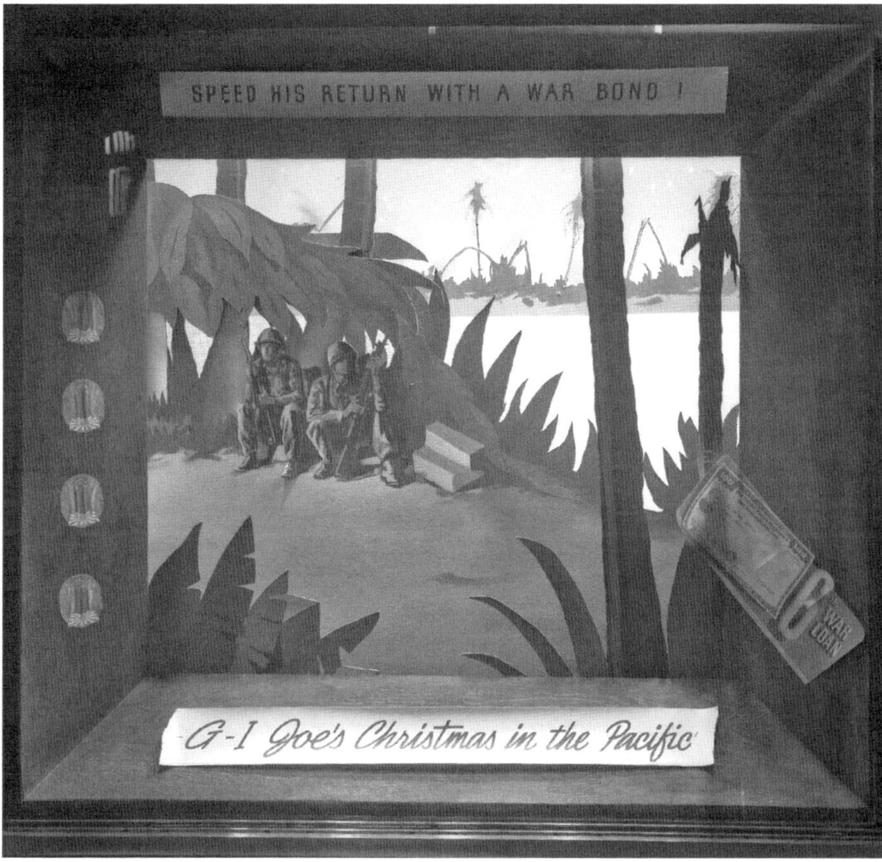

War bond window display at the Vic Hanny Company, a local Phoenix men's clothing store. The caption reads: "SPEED HIS RETURN WITH A WAR BOND!" The display depicts GI Joe's Christmas in the Pacific. *McCulloch Brothers Inc. Photographs, CP MCLMB. Arizona State University Libraries: Arizona Collection.*

continent. The Irish migrated to Arizona earlier in the twentieth century seeking work in the mining industry and a better life. Sovereign Native American nations occupied a quarter of the state's area. With World War II came an influx of enemy Germans and Italians, as well as Americans of Japanese descent. Cadet nurses in Arizona trained in a volatile context during this wartime emergency.

In this context, the state- and local-level affiliates of the National Nursing Council for War Service made a concentrated effort to attract volunteers for service in the U.S. Cadet Nurse Corps. Qualified volunteers would apply for admission to any of the state's five hospital schools of nursing.

Chapter 3

HOSPITAL SCHOOLS OF NURSING IN ARIZONA

Arizona's five participating schools of nursing in the U.S. Cadet Nurse Corps were at Sage Memorial, Saint Mary's, Santa Monica's, Saint Joseph's and Good Samaritan Hospitals. Saint Mary's in Tucson trained the largest number and Sage Memorial in Ganado on the Navajo Reservation the fewest. Saint Joseph's Hospital School of Nursing was the oldest in the state, and Santa Monica's the youngest. Good Samaritan Hospital School of Nursing was originally known as Deaconess Hospital. All five schools had religious roots, and each had a unique mission and history.

Sage Memorial Hospital School of Nursing

Sage Memorial Hospital School of Nursing, located in Ganado, Arizona, was the nation's only accredited school of nursing for Native Americans. The hospital and school of nursing operated from 1930 to 1953. Though over time, the school of nursing extended its scope to include Hispanic and Asian students, it unapologetically excluded white students. White students, it was reported, had many options from which to choose, but Native Americans did not.

Dr. Clarence Salsbury was the superintendent, medical director and chief surgeon of Sage Memorial (also known as the Ganado Mission of

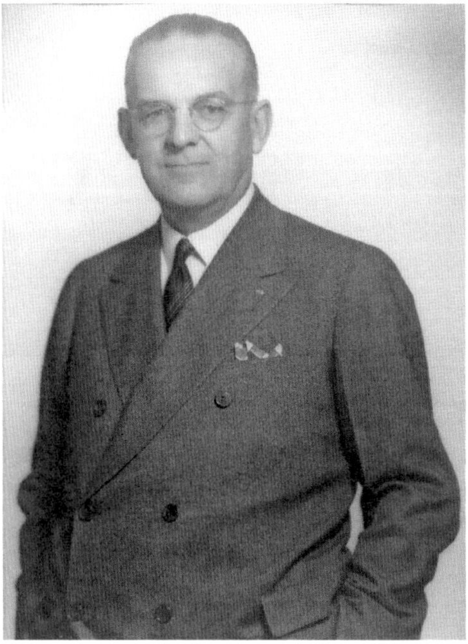

Dr. Clarence Salsbury, superintendent, Sage Memorial Hospital. *Arizona State Library.*

the Presbyterian Church). Dr. Salsbury was Canadian by birth and trained for medical missionary work in Brooklyn, New York. His first mission was in China. Sage Memorial was his second mission. He arrived in Ganado in 1927 with his wife, Cora, who was a nurse. He remained at Sage Memorial until 1950. In 1951, he was appointed state of Arizona commissioner of health welfare and in 1952 took the position of commissioner of public health for the state of Arizona.

Sage Memorial Hospital was dedicated on May 14, 1930. It was the most advanced medical facility on the Navajo Reservation with seventy-five beds, a surgical unit, laboratory, X-ray department and modern kitchen. It is said that the impressive structure enabled Salisbury to recruit additional physicians and launch an ambitious healthcare program. By the end of the New Deal era, Sage Memorial Hospital's and Salsbury's presence could not be ignored.[22]

Although a goal of the hospital was to improve the quality of healthcare on the reservation, its main goal was unapologetic religious indoctrination and conversion. Student nurses were expected to give up their private lives along with much of their cultural identity.[23] Salsbury was also convinced that Navajos would respond better to Native American nurses, who would understand patients better as well as operate an understaffed hospital inexpensively. For these reasons, he decided to open a school of nursing. This effort was met with some tribal opposition to women leaving home to pursue a career, and Salsbury enlisted the aid of tribal leadership to build trust among the Navajo community and overcome some of the skepticism.[24] Indian Service officials also warned Dr. Salsbury that the school would fail. The school of nursing received full accreditation from the Arizona State Board of Nursing Examiners in January 1932. The school of nursing flourished.

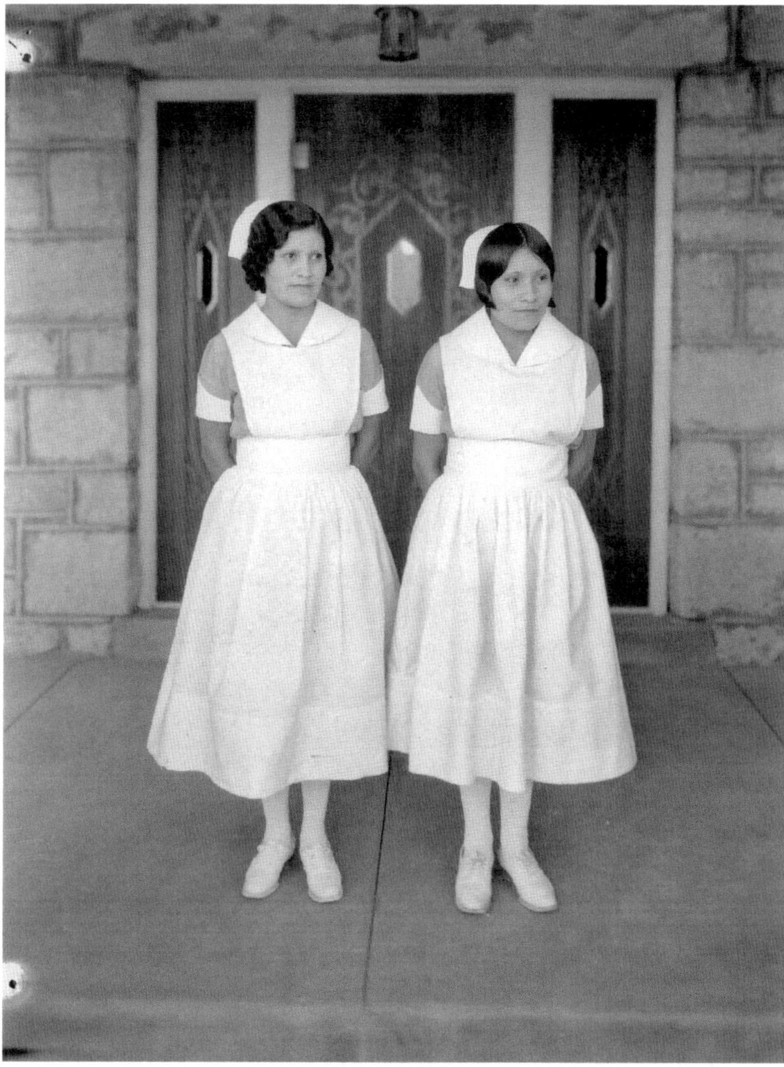

Adele Slivers (left) and Ruth Henderson are commemorated here as the first graduates from the Sage Memorial Hospital School of Nursing in Ganado, Arizona, on November 29, 1933. At the time, it served as the only accredited School of Nursing for Native American women. They were also the first Navajo women to come before the Arizona State Board of Nurse Examiners on October 20–21, 1933. *Arizona Historical Society Library and Archives, Tempe.*

Adele Slivers and Ruth Henderson were Sage Memorial's first graduates to pass the Arizona State Boards in 1933. Slivers, the daughter of a Native American medicine man, would work at Sage Memorial in the surgical department and later report to Albuquerque Air Base in New Mexico as a second lieutenant in the Army Nurse Corps Reserves during World War II. She was "on the front lines between modern medicine and Navajo tradition."[25]

During World War II, Sage Memorial Hospital began to experience the same shortage of nurses experienced in hospitals across the country at that time. Sage cadet nurses, such as Rowena Pentawa and Alyce Valandry, served and were recognized by the community for their service. They also represented the corps at the launching of a ship in California. The July 23, 1945 *Prescott Courier* carried this news story:

> *Cadet Nurses Alyce Valandry and Rowena Pentewa of Sage Memorial Hospital, Ganado, Arizona, largest Indian hospital in the Southwest, are greeted by Chief Richard Davis Thunderbird, priest chief of the Dog*

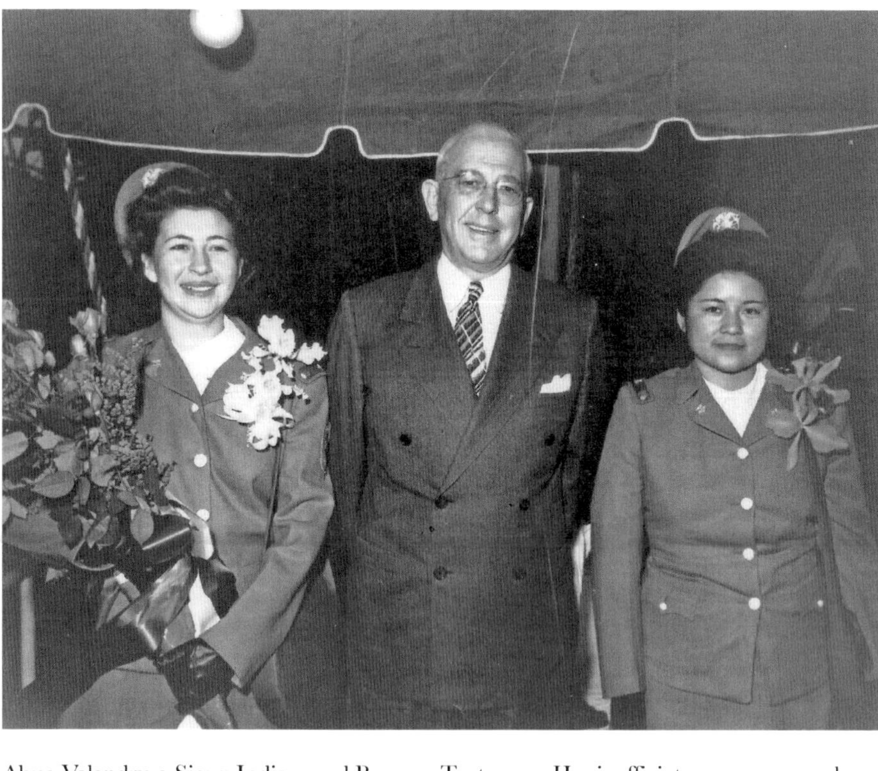

Alyce Valandry, a Sioux Indian, and Rowena Tentewa, a Hopi, officiate as sponsor and maid of honor at the launching of SS *Coastal Nomad* at the Consolidated Steel Company Shipyards in Wilmington, California, on July 9, 1945. Both cadets are from Sage Memorial School of Nursing in Ganado, Arizona. *National Archives and Records Administration.*

> *Soldiers band of the Cheyenne Indians, on their arrival in Los Angeles recently via Santa Fe Railway's California Limited. Enrolled in the* [C]*adet* [N]*urse* [C]*orps of the U.S. Public Health Service, the Indian nurses journeyed to the Coast to participate in launching of the M.S.* Coastal Nomad, *war cargo vessel, at the Wilmington yards of the Consolidated Steel Corp*[oration]. *Nurse Valandry was sponsor of the vessel, Nurse Pentewa was maid of honor, and chief Thunderbird performed an Indian Good Luck ceremony for the ship.*

The story also ran in the *Cadet Nurse Corps News*, a Public Health Service newsletter with national readership.

After 1945, with nursing education moving into the universities, practical training obtained at Sage became less useful in passing state exams as nursing requirements began to emphasize college curriculum. Also, racial barriers in the United States were beginning to lower, making alternative programs available to Native Americans. After Salsbury's retirement in 1950 came a reassessment of the school of nursing and the decision to close the registered nursing program and replacing it with a curriculum in practical nursing. The final class of registered nurses graduated in 1951: Cecelia Lauriano (Sandia Pueblo), Margaret Lujan (Taos), Elaine Abraham (Thlinget), Lydia

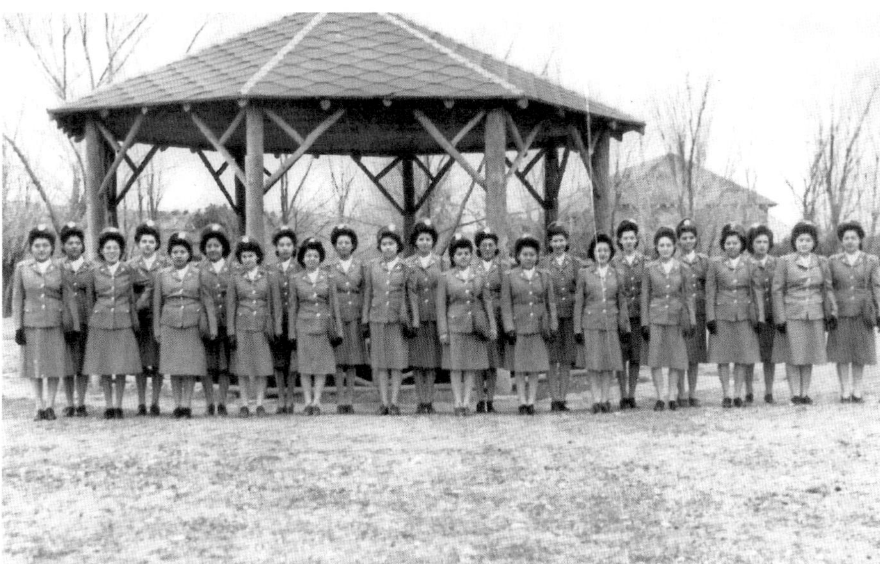

Native American cadet nurses, Sage Memorial School of Nursing. *National Archive and Records Administration.*

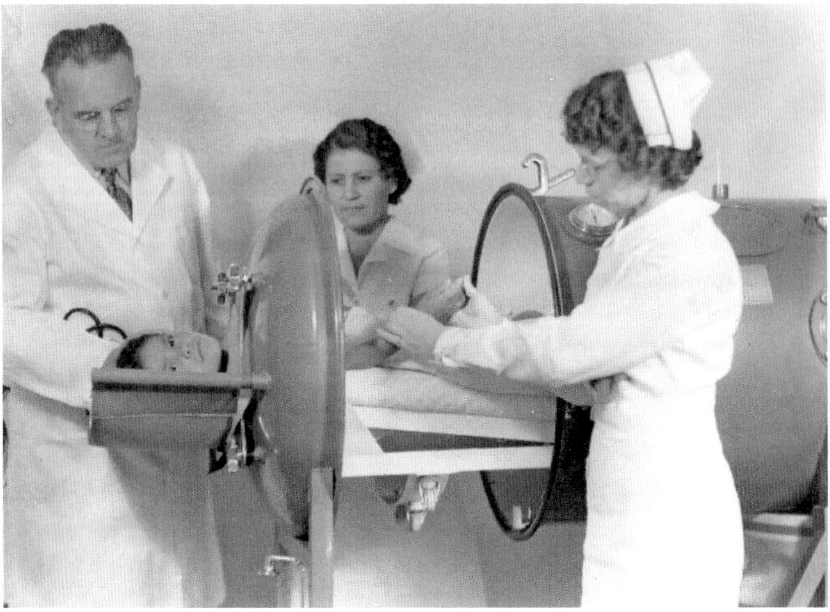

Photograph of Dr. Clarence Salsbury and nurses using an iron lung with a young girl at the Sage Memorial Hospital in Ganado, Arizona, circa 1945. *Arizona State Library, Archives and Public Records.*

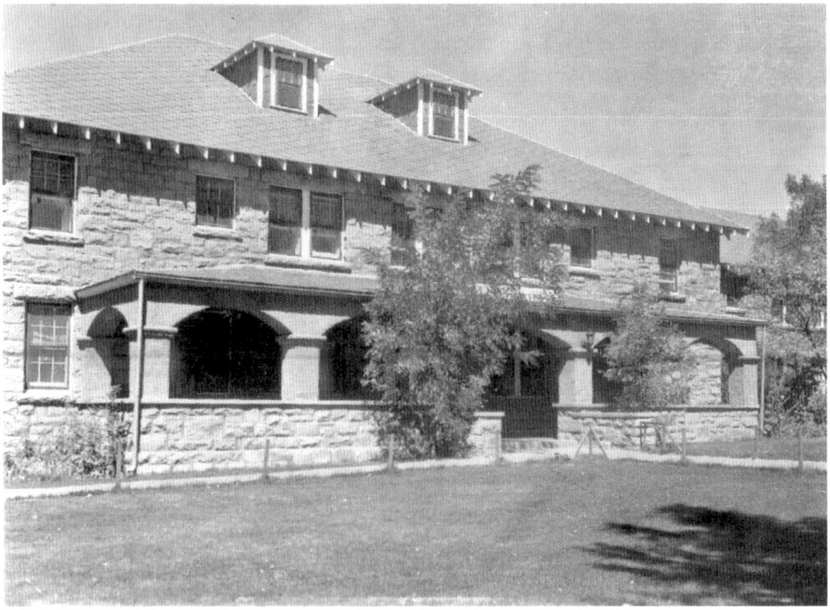

Photograph of Sage Memorial Hospital at the Ganado Presbyterian Mission in Ganado, Arizona, circa 1940. *Arizona State Library, Archives and Public Records.*

Bear (Winnebago), Janet Begay (Navajo), Birdie Collier (Philippines) and Susie Esquibel (Spanish American).

Over the course of its two decades, Viola García, a Sage Memorial graduate, reported that the Sage Memorial Hospital School of Nursing graduated about 150 native women from more than fifty tribes.[26] Among those women were 39 Cadet Nurses.[27] Although forced to jettison most of their cultural heritage, Sage Memorial graduates received high praise from the Anglo community and proved conclusively that Native American women were capable of meeting high academic standards and working effectively in the medical profession. They also brought medical care to people in need, a commitment to service that some say has yet to be fully appreciated.

GOOD SAMARITAN HOSPITAL SCHOOL OF NURSING

Arizona Deaconess Hospital was established by Lulu Clifton, a Methodist deaconess who arrived in Phoenix in 1911 to recuperate from tuberculosis. She was convinced that Phoenix needed a new hospital. Her first hospital facility was located in an apartment building in downtown Phoenix. Later she leased an office building from a doctor. In 1917, Clifton and her supporters acquired a square block of donated land along McDowell Road, which at that time was considered to be out in the country. A new 105-bed hospital with five operating rooms was built on this land and opened in 1923. This new facility also had a special obstetrical delivery unit and Arizona's first incubator. In 1928, the hospital's name was changed to Good Samaritan Hospital.

The nursing school opened in 1920. The purpose of the nursing school was to "establish, maintain and conduct a Christian School of Nursing for the proper training of young women as nurses." Students were admitted in September 1920. By 1928, the minimum entrance requirements for the thirty-month-long school of nursing program were being age eighteen and having at least three years of high school. The school was accredited in 1925 by the Arizona State Board of Examiners. The School of Nursing was reported to have introduced higher entrance requirements by 1946, likely a result of participation in the U.S. Cadet Nurse Corps, when students had to be seventeen years old and have completed four years of high school. There was a six-month preclinical period, and total course was thirty-six months. Over the course of its fifty-three-year history, Good Samaritan Hospital School of Nursing prepared

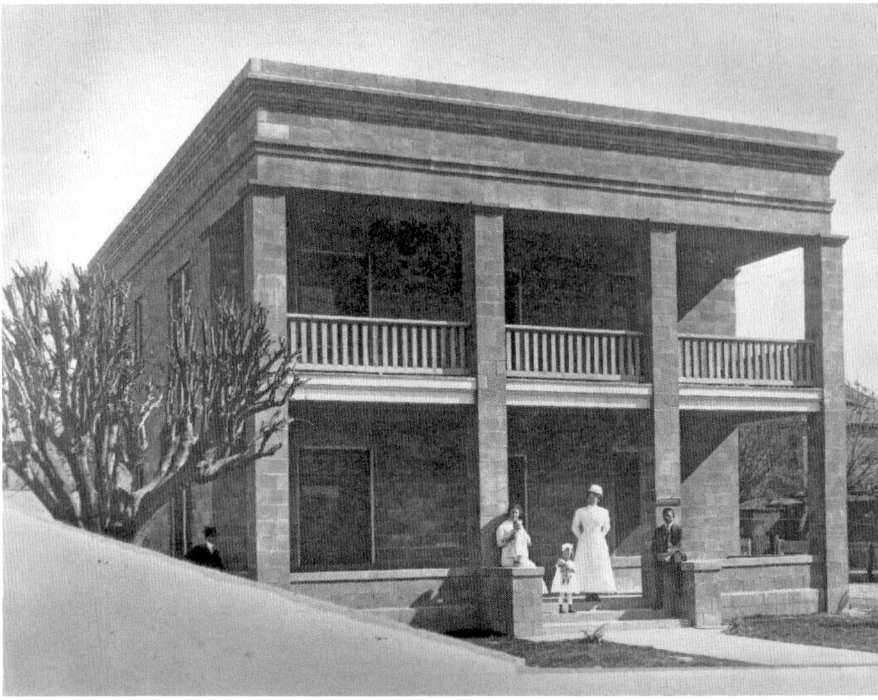

Original Deaconess Hospital in downtown Phoenix, 1911–14. *Courtesy of Banner-University Medical Center, Phoenix, Arizona.*

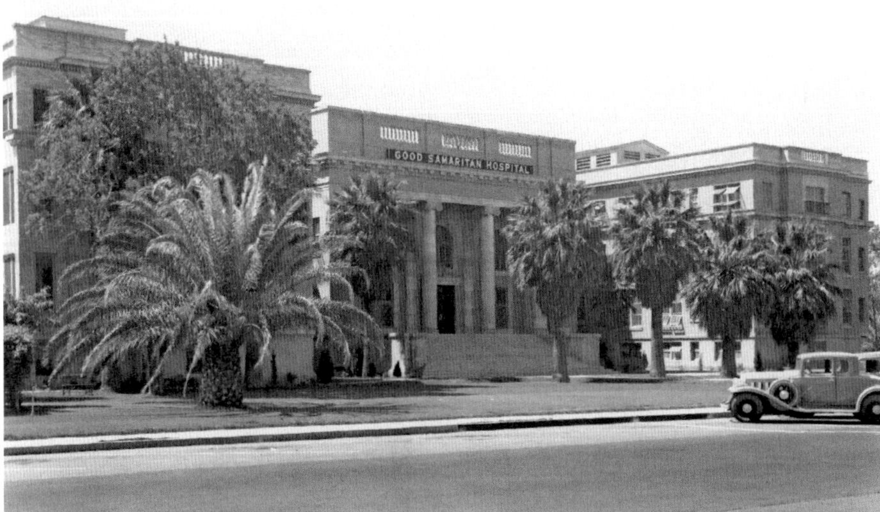

Good Samaritan Hospital, 1924. *Courtesy of Banner-University Medical Center, Phoenix, Arizona.*

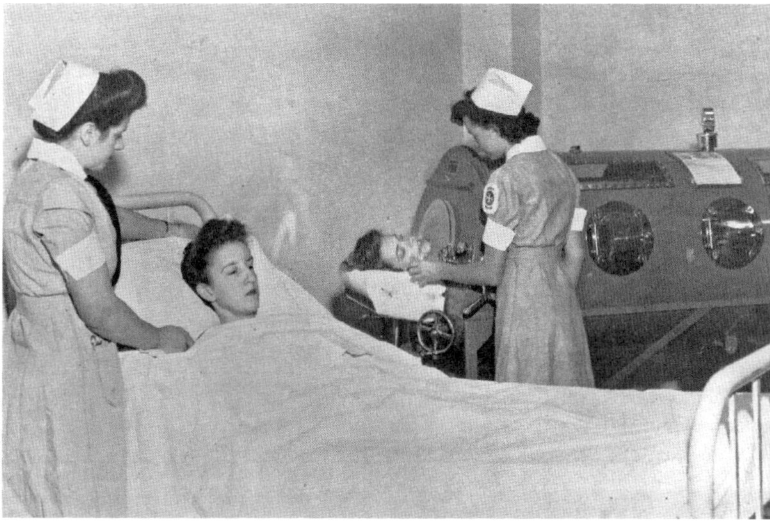

"Nurses with Polio Patients at Good Samaritan Hospital." A cadet nurse tending to a polio patient in an iron lung. The iron lung was one of a number of medical innovations introduced during and shortly after World War II. *Courtesy of Banner-University Medical Center, Phoenix, Arizona.*

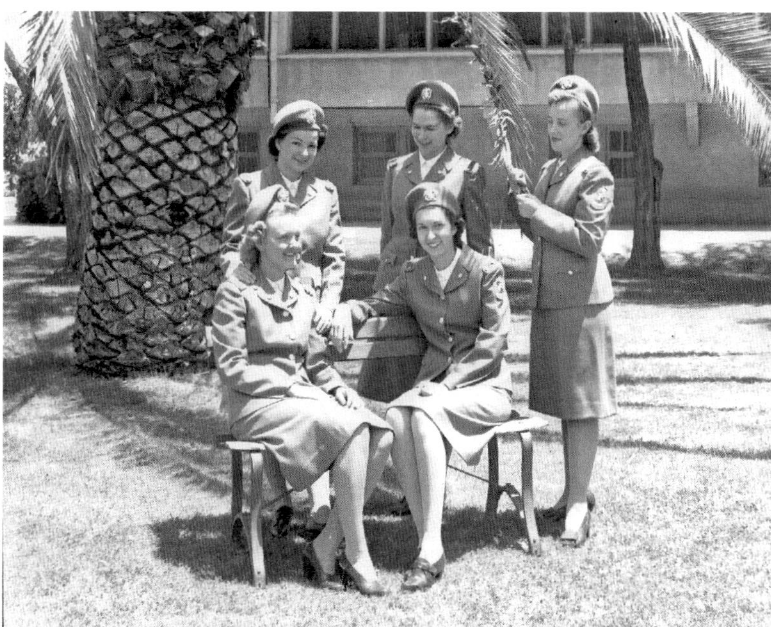

Above and next page: Good Samaritan Hospital School of Nursing cadet nurses in uniform. *National Archives and Records Administration.*

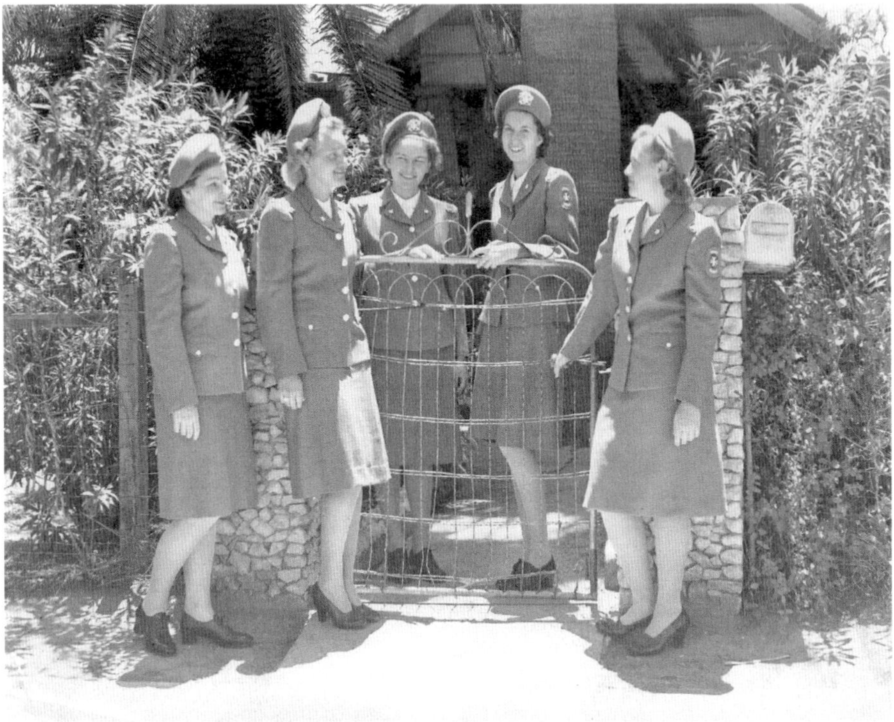

1,400 young women to be nurses, including Janet Lowe, the hospital's first baby girl born at the hospital, in 1923. Janet was the daughter of a nurse, and she was a cadet nurse at Good Samaritan. Good Samaritan School of Nursing closed in 1973.

SAINT JOSEPH'S HOSPITAL SCHOOL OF NURSING

Formal nurse education came to Arizona for the first time at the state's oldest nursing school at Saint Joseph's Hospital in Phoenix. In 1895, the hospital was established in an adobe house located at Polk and Fourth Streets in what is now downtown Phoenix. The Catholic Sisters of Mercy created it as a tuberculosis sanatorium for six patients. Doctors came to this hospital by horse and buggy and on bicycles. As the population grew, so did the hospital. A new section was added in 1911. It later developed into a 140-bed hospital. A fire destroyed the hospital in 1917, but it was rebuilt quickly. This new building, opened in 1927, was reported in the *Arizona Republican* newspaper to be "most complete, scientific, and modern in its equipment as any in the Southwest." People of all races and religions were welcome at Saint Joseph's, regardless of ability to pay.

The sisters arrived in Arizona in 1892 to educate children, not to provide healthcare, but they soon discovered a great need for the latter. Saint Joseph's Hospital in Phoenix was one of a number of hospitals in Arizona that they managed. The sisters were also recognized intercultural brokers; they learned Spanish; celebrated the feast of Our Lady of Guadalupe, a Mexican saint; and served as a bridge between the different cultures coexisting in Phoenix.[28]

With the dawn of the twentieth century came a move toward the professionalization of medicine and nursing. The Saint Joseph's Hospital Nurse Training School opened in 1910 with a standardized curriculum that predated national standards for nurse education, which would appear four years later. Though not the oldest hospital in the state (Saint Mary's Hospital in Tucson was established in 1880), Saint Joseph's Hospital School of Nursing occupies the distinction of being the first school of nursing in Arizona.

According to Dora Burch, who was a student at Saint Joseph's Training School in 1915:

> *The entrance requirement then was one year of high school or its equivalent. Most of the girls were very young—16 or 17 years old. In our class, I*

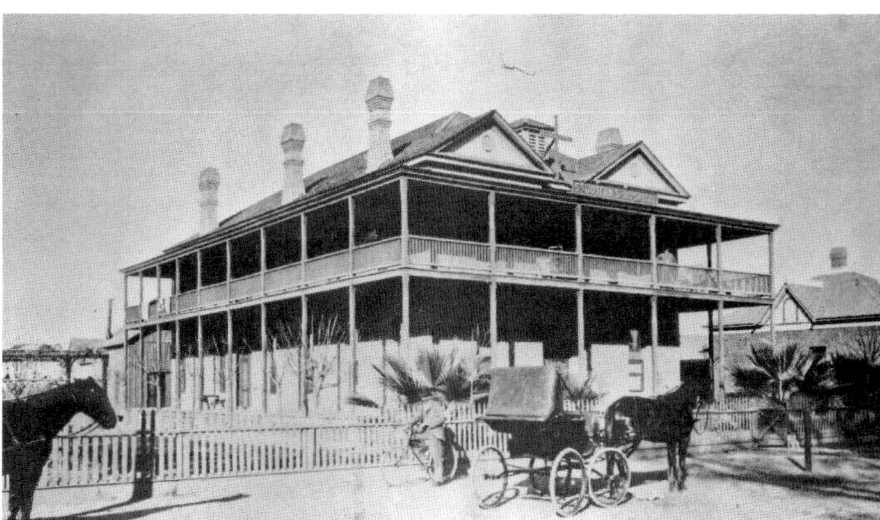

Saint Joseph's Hospital, 1905. *Arizona State Library.*

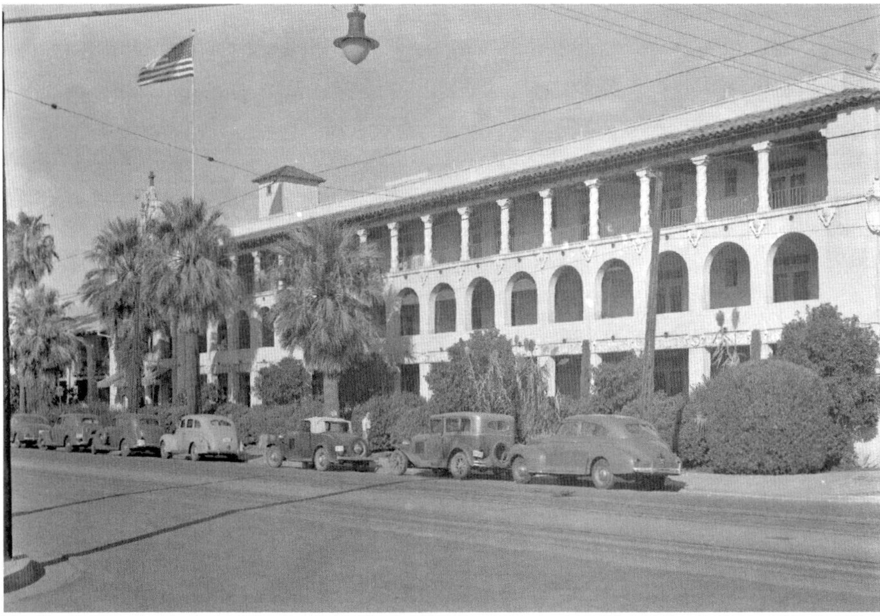

Saint Joseph's Hospital, circa 1941. *McCulloch Brothers Inc. Photographs, CP MCLMB A1256A. Arizona State University Libraries: Arizona Collection.*

> *remember, about fifteen entered the same time I did. Only four finished. Besides me, there were Sister M. Bertram, Sister M. Genevieve, and Elizabeth McClellan.*
>
> *Classes were taught by Sisters and doctors. Nursing techniques were taught on the wards. Doctors taught anatomy; physiology; surgery; communicable disease; obstetrics; bacteriology; and eye, ear, nose and throat.*[29]

By 1928, admissions requirements had changed: entering nursing students had to be eighteen years old and have four years of high school. Student nurses worked forty-eight hours a week exclusive of classes. The course was thirty months long. Student nurses received small monthly stipends.

In 1946, there were 119 students. During World War II, nearly 200 student nurses at Saint Joseph's were cadet nurses. Saint Joseph's Hospital School of Nursing closed in 1970.

SANTA MONICA'S HOSPITAL SCHOOL OF NURSING

Santa Monica's Hospital in South Phoenix, Arizona, was part of a federally funded community development project spearheaded by Emmett McLoughlin, who was a Franciscan priest. Santa Monica's was the first integrated hospital and interracial school of nursing west of the Mississippi River. Its aim was to

> *provide the best possible nursing training and experience to young women regardless of their racial or religious background. This is based on the American and Christian doctrine that all men are created equal and should have equal opportunities. Santa Monica's is the first nurses' training school in the history of the United States to open its doors with this definite policy.*[30]

Father Emmett moved to Southwest Phoenix in the 1930s. The densely populated area was outside the Phoenix city limits at the time. It was a fringe area located between the warehouse district and the city dump. Dwellings were, for the most part, without electricity and many without plumbing and heat. Poverty and disease were part of everyday life. There was an acute lack of health services, especially maternity services. During these early days, Father Emmett established a church and community center in a remodeled grocery store and in 1934 opened Arizona's first maternity clinic.

In 1938, Franklin Delano Roosevelt reported that one-third of the nation was ill clothed, ill fed and ill housed. This statement was painfully true in Phoenix. Father Emmett argued for public housing, which ultimately led to the establishment of federally funded housing in South Phoenix.

With World War II came another healthcare challenge in Arizona in the form of venereal disease among the influx of military personnel and defense workers at nearby Luke Airfield. The promiscuous women of Phoenix were blamed for the outbreak of syphilis among air force soldiers stationed at the base. Phoenix health authorities replied that the air force was "contaminating the purity of Phoenix womanhood."[31] The army ultimately ordered all of Phoenix off-limits to military personnel. This influx of military personnel and defense workers strained healthcare facilities in the Valley, and the poor minorities in Southwest Phoenix were often the last to receive medical treatment.

However, the incidence of venereal disease—which caused a rift in the community—was also an impetus for the development of a new hospital for this underserved portion of South Phoenix. At the time, when the Board of Santa Monica's sought property for its planned fifty-bed hospital, a new federal ruling required that all community facilities financed under the Lanham Act be approved by the War Department. The nearest War Department representative to Phoenix was the same air field administered by those who complained about Phoenix's loose women. Father Emmett met with the commanding officer at Luke Field, who agreed to support this building project under the condition that the hospital capacity be doubled and that half the beds be reserved for the treatment of venereal disease. On August 10, 1942, Father Emmett received word that the president of the United States approved funding for the hospital.

In 1943, the 232-bed community-based medical Santa Monica's Hospital facility was built and dedicated to caring for the community regardless of ethnic origin or socioeconomic status. On February 14, 1944, the new hospital opened its doors to the first patient, and on October 1, 1944, the nursing school opened. With Santa Monica's School of Nursing's opening began its participation in the newly established U.S. Cadet Nurse Corps. Santa Monica's Hospital and School of Nursing were located in what was considered a "slum area" of South Phoenix.[32]

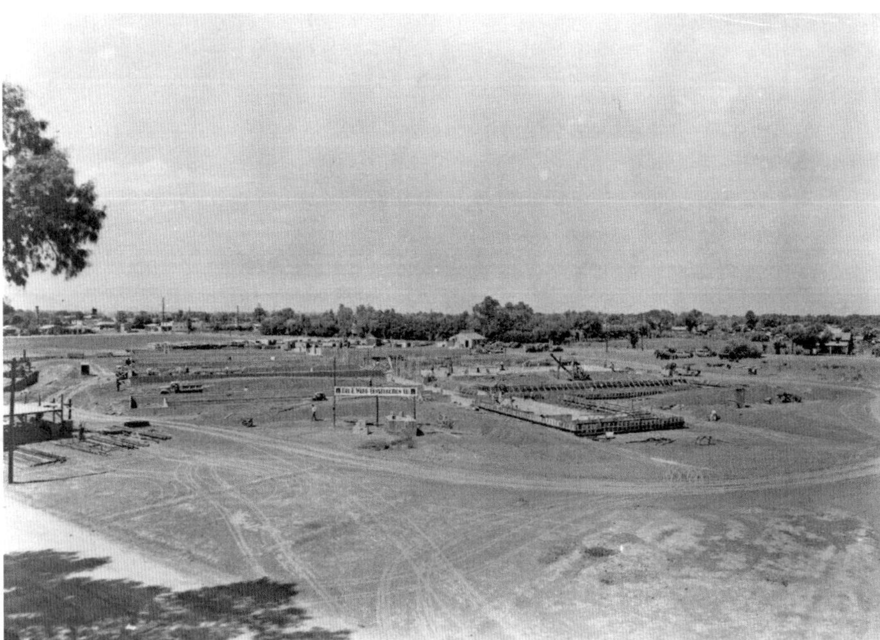

Santa Monica's (Memorial) Hospital under construction in 1942. The hospital was built on what had been previously the center of a cotton field in south Phoenix. *Herb and Dorothy McLaughlin Photographs, Arizona State University Libraries.*

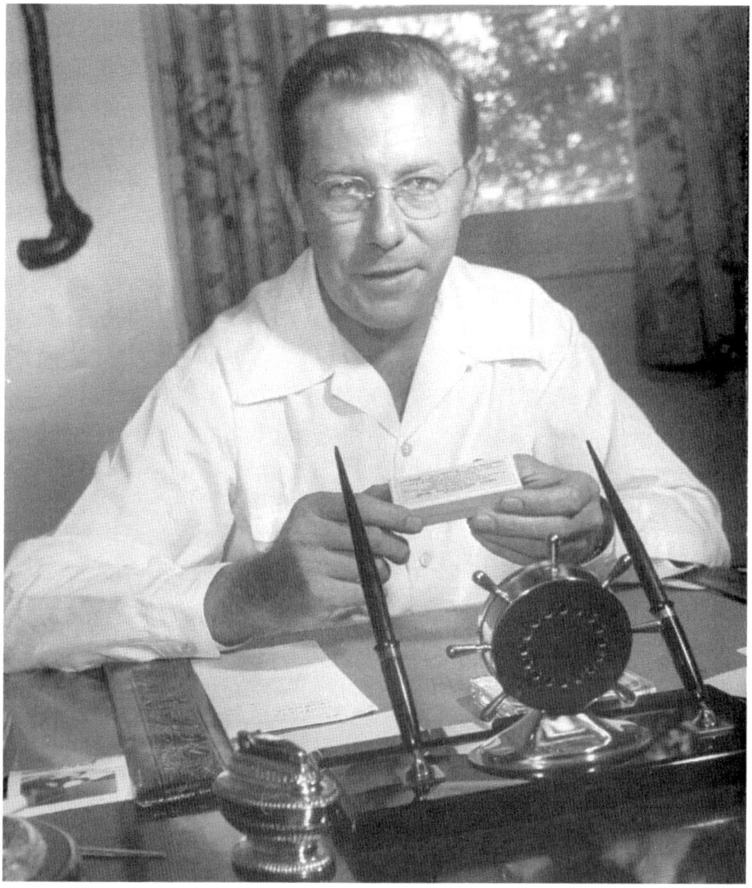

Emmett McLoughlin, superintendent, Santa Monica's Hospital. McLoughlin is holding contraband scorpion anti-venom medication, smuggled into the United States from Mexico. He is said to have encouraged the use of this medication at Santa Monica's because it worked better than medication available in the United States. This photo was taken in 1945. *Peter Stackpole/The LIFE Picture Collection/Getty Images.*

McLoughlin's secular activities frequently met with disapproval from his superiors. Dubbed "America's most famous ex-priest," he left the priesthood after the war, in 1948, to remain superintendent of Santa Monica's Hospital (later known as Phoenix Memorial Hospital). Before World War II, he was instrumental in securing federal funds for three public housing projects: the Marcos de Niza Project for Mexicans, the Matthew Henson Project for blacks (both located in South Phoenix) and the Frank Luke Jr. Project for Anglos, located in East Phoenix. He was appointed as the first chairman of the Phoenix Housing Authority in 1939, and served as secretary of the Arizona State Board of Health. McLoughlin established a policy of treating all Santa Monica's patients, regardless of ability to pay. He established the state's first polio ward, and to prevent needless deaths from scorpion stings, he encouraged the smuggling of anti-venom medication into Phoenix from Mexico in blatant violation of federal law.

Father Emmett had once asked nearby Saint Joseph's Hospital School of Nursing officials to accept a black student, but they refused. When Mrs. Roosevelt visited Father Emmett at Santa Monica's Hospital after the war, she wrote that she was "particularly interested in the training school for nurses. Here they have eliminated all discrimination of race and color. They all study and work together. The hospital has a wonderful atmosphere."[33] Mrs. Roosevelt noted its wonderful, interracial atmosphere, where everyone worked together.

In a news story on the graduation of the second interracial class that appeared in the *Arizona Republic* newspaper on June 27, 1948, it was also reported that Saint Luke's Hospital in Spokane, Washington, had been studying Santa Monica's integrated model and was going to follow it the following year in its school of nursing. Following this policy would demonstrate that Saint Luke's in no way condoned racial prejudices. Said Father Emmett: "If the young people of the nation adopt this attitude, there is no need to worry too much about intolerance in the future." In the last class of cadet nurses at Santa Monica's were three African Americans, one Spanish American and one Sioux Indian. The March 7, 1945 *Phoenix Gazette* reported on another Santa Monica student, Cyrilla Endfield, of the San Carlos Apache community, which is about one hundred miles east of Phoenix. She was on a shopping trip in Phoenix with her mother and sister, a private in the Women's Army Corps. Their mother, Goldie Endfield, was pictured in traditional native dress and flanked by her two daughters, each in her respective uniform.

Santa Monica's was known as a haven "for all races" and had evolved into Phoenix Memorial Hospital by 1951. In the 1950s, its reputation as "the hospital with a heart" increased. McLoughlin remained superintendent of Memorial Hospital until his death in 1970. The School of Nursing closed in 1956. During its twelve years' existence, Santa Monica's graduated between 98 and 145 nurses.[34]

Saint Mary's Hospital School of Nursing

Saint Mary's Hospital, located in Tucson, Arizona, is the oldest hospital in Arizona. It was founded in 1880 by Bishop Jean-Baptiste Salpointe and sold to the Sisters of Saint Joseph of Carondelet, a teaching order, in 1882, provided that it remain a hospital.

The school of nursing was established in 1914. Sister Mary Fidelia McMahon planned the school of nursing, and Sisters Francis de Sales Fuller and Mary Evangelista Weyand were transferred to Tucson from Kansas City, Missouri, to prepare the curriculum and organize a teaching faculty. The curriculum at Saint Mary's included subject areas like anatomy and physiology, methods of nursing, materia medica, ethics, dietetics, obstetrics and gynecology, hygiene, bacteriology, urinalysis, pediatrics, contagious diseases, surgical nursing and first aid. This curriculum predated the publication of the first national curriculum norms, *The Standard Curriculum for Schools of Nursing*[35] by three years.

The first class of Saint Mary's Hospital School of Nursing graduated in 1917. Sister Evangelista assisted in preparing a bill for the state legislature to empower Governor Thomas Campbell to appoint a State Board of Nursing Examiners "to regulate professional nursing in the state of Arizona, providing for the examination and the issuing of certificates to graduate nurses, and providing penalty for the violation of the act." This original law was binding until 1952, when a new law was passed that provided for the Arizona State Board of Nurse Registration and Nurse Education.

Sister Evangelista was charter member of the Arizona State Board of Nursing Examiners in the 1920s and recognized as registered nurse No. 1, the first licensed registered nurse in Arizona.[36] She also was a founder of the Arizona State Nurses Association and is credited with raising professional standards for nursing and nurse education in the West.

In June 1943, the U.S. Cadet Nurse Corps was established at Saint Mary's. During the first six months of the program, Sister Mary Beatrice Johnson, director of the school, enrolled fifty-four students in the corps. In addition to the two classes annually received into the school, January and September, a class was accepted in June 1944. The cadets enrolled at the University of Arizona for the regular course of chemistry; the limited facilities of the school could not accommodate the large classes. The auxiliary of the Pima County Medical Society assisted by providing transportation for the students to and from the university.

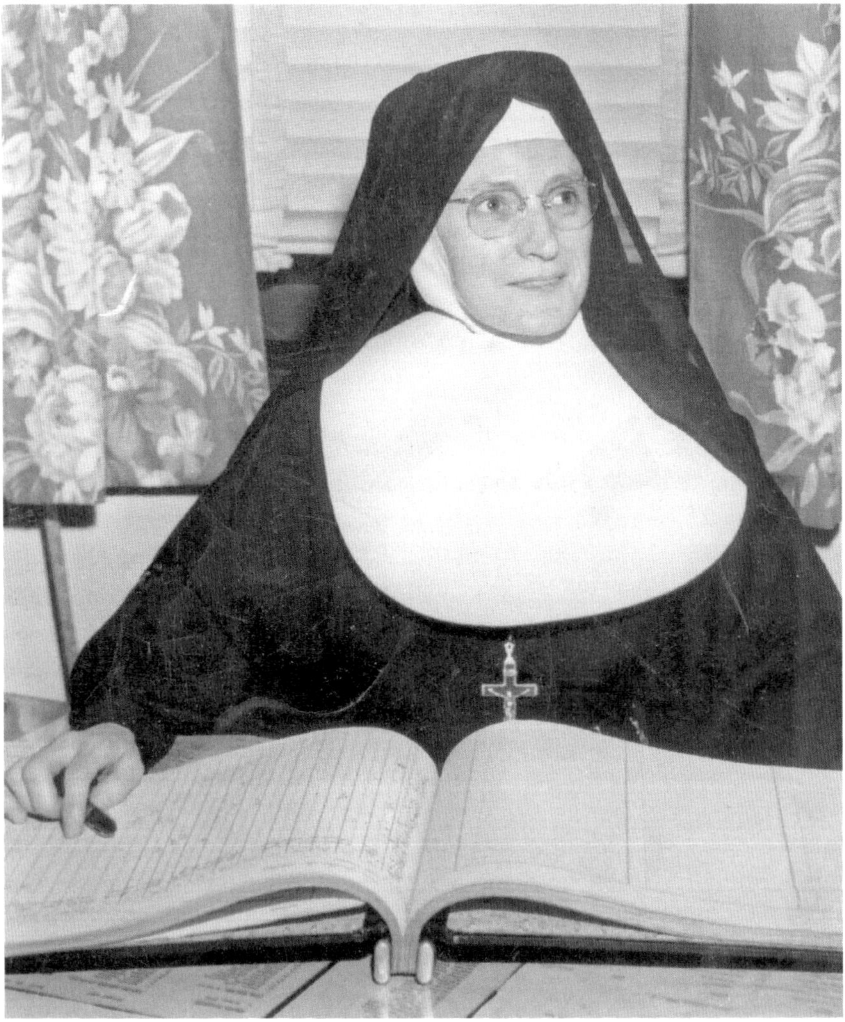

Sister Beatrice Johnson administered Saint Mary's School of Nursing during the 1940s. *Courtesy of Sisters of St. Joseph of Carondelet, Los Angeles Province Archives.*

The local press was generous in presenting material recommended or prepared by the school. In one article, Constance Campioni, science instructor at Saint Mary's School of Nursing wrote: "We at Saint Mary's are looking ahead to the post-war world which is certain to be handicapped by disease, malnutrition and other enemies of health brought on by the conflict. The need will be there. We hope that we can do our small part in providing the trained help which will be necessary."[37]

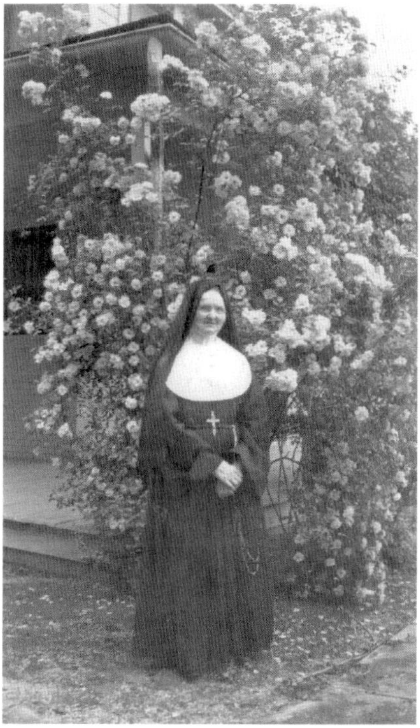

Right: Sister Mary Evangelista Weyand developed St. Mary's School of Nursing and was Arizona's first registered nurse. *Courtesy of Sisters of St. Joseph of Carondelet, Los Angeles Province Archives.*

Below: Cadet nurses visit Marana Air Field in 1945 accompanied by their instructor, Miss Lubeck. The Marana Air Field was one of the many military installations in Arizona. *Courtesy of Sisters of St. Joseph of Carondelet, Los Angeles Province Archives.*

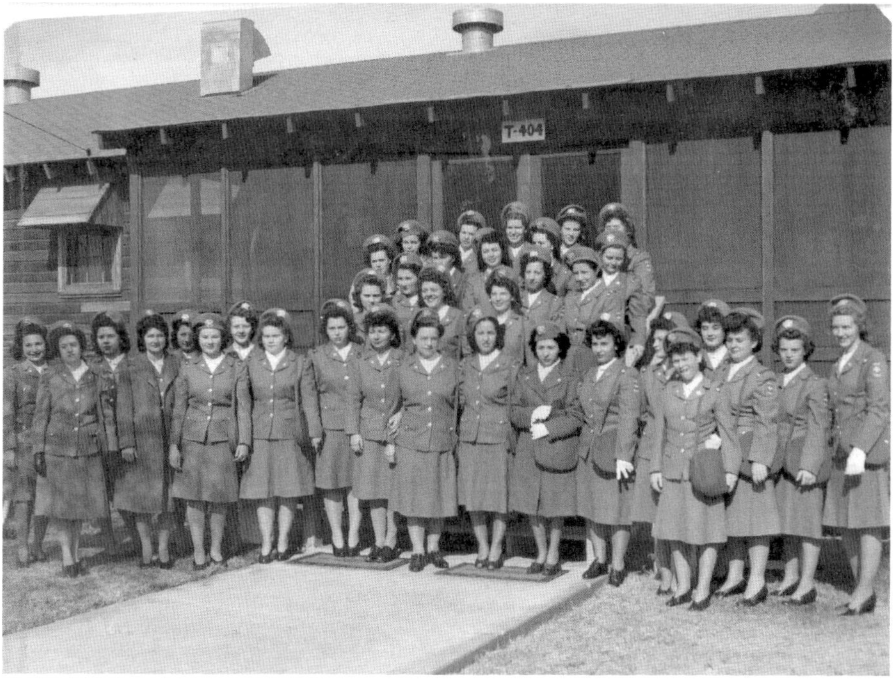

Saint Mary's Hospital School of Nursing closed in 1966, a casualty of financial pressure and the realization that nurse education had changed and the movement from hospital-based training to college education to prepare nurses was complete.

Chapter 4

ARIZONA'S CADET NURSES

In this chapter, we explore two groups of cadet nurses who lived in Arizona. One group includes some 710 women who were trained in Arizona's five participating schools of nursing during World War II; the other group consists of 25 women who were cadet nurses elsewhere in the United States during World War II and were living in Arizona in the 1980s. Through an exploration of archival evidence—cadet nurse membership cards of those trained in Arizona and the transcripts of 25 cadet nurses who were interviewed toward the end of their careers in the late 1980s—we will glean some general impressions about their backgrounds and experiences. Of particular interest are these nurses' training experiences during World War II, the degree to which ethnic and racial minorities participated in this program, and retrospective interpretations on the importance of the Cadet Nurse Corps program on their careers and personal lives.

Training Experiences During World War II

To gain insight into Cadet Nurses in Arizona, I collected their membership cards from the National Archives and transcribed card data into a spreadsheet for descriptive analysis.[38] There were 710 Arizona cadet nurse membership cards in the database. Thirty-eight percent were eighteen years old or younger, and over half were between nineteen and twenty-nine years

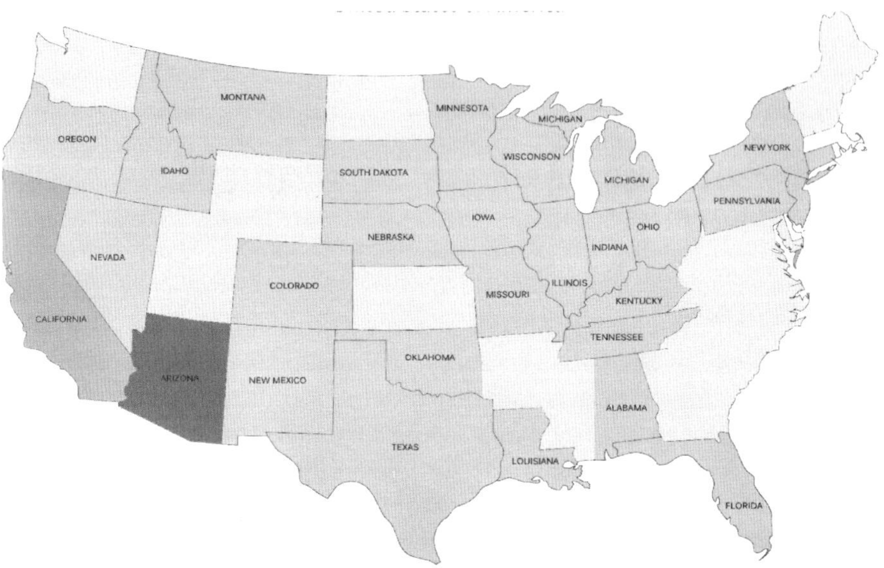

Map of the United States showing the states of origin of cadet nurses trained in Arizona. The darker the state is shaded, the more cadet nurses the state sent to Arizona schools. *Illustration by author.*

old. Less than 3 percent were thirty years old or older. They came from thirty states. Over 50 percent were from Arizona and nearly 11 percent from California. That so many came from the East and the Plains states may be attributable to the economic situation at the time. The cadet nurses of the 1940s were the children of the 1930s, and many migrated with their families across the country in search of work after the Great Depression. Also among the membership cards was one showing the hometown of the student as Cananea, Sonora, Mexico, a mining town not too far from the mines in southern Arizona.

Cadet nurses in these schools of nursing were of modest means, according to their reports of their fathers', guardians' or spouses' occupations. One hundred forty-three cadet nurses reported a parent, guardian or spouse who worked in agriculture, ranching or the mining industry, which were common occupations in Arizona at the time. Nineteen reported a retired or deceased parent, guardian or spouse. The occupation of the parent, guardian or spouse of 29 of the cadet nurses was reported as housewife, reflecting possibly that a male breadwinner was not present in the household. Sixty-seven cadet nurses reported parents, guardians or spouses in the military or government work, and 48 were reported as professionals, such as teachers, civil engineers, physicians, judges or clergy members. The cadet nurses reported 47 parents, guardians or spouses who were carpenters, plumbers or electricians. Eighty-six were small business owners, such as bakers, grocers, restaurateurs, realtors or other businesses not necessarily related to the defense industry. Another 129 were reported as working in some sort of manufacturing occupation that appeared related to the defense industry. Twenty-two were reported as clerical workers or laborers.

Finally, thirty fathers, guardians or spouses were reported as working in some capacity with the railroad, generally the Southern Pacific Railroad. Other employers mentioned were two mining companies: the Miami (Arizona) Copper Company and the Phelps-Dodge Corporation. A number of companies related to the defense industry were also reported: the Ford Motor Company, the Goodyear Air Corporation, the Quincy (Illinois) Barge Company and the Ryan School of Aeronautics. Other employers were the Wisconsin Bell Telephone Company, JCPenney and Standard Oil. Government-related employers included the U.S. Internal Revenue Service, the Tucson (Arizona) Police Department and the War Production Board of Arizona,

Of the 710 cadet nurses' membership cards, 381, or 54.0 percent, graduated and became licensed nurses. Approximately 46.0 percent, or 325, withdrew from the program, and one died in training. This rate of withdrawal compares unfavorably with the national withdrawal rates for 1944, 1945 and 1946 of 39.2, 39.4 and 30.8 percent, respectively.[39] Nationally, academic failure accounted for only 24.0 percent of withdrawals by cadet nurses from nursing school. Students also withdrew because of failure to meet other standards, marriage, health, maladjustment and loss of interest, other personal reasons, family needs or no reason given. The membership cards do not indicate the reason for Arizona cadet nurses' withdrawal from the program, but one might conjecture that a similar proportion of Arizona's cadet nurses withdrew for academic reasons, as well.

Diversity Among Students Trained in Arizona

The membership card data did not include an indication of the students' race or ethnicity, which makes it difficult to assess the diversity of the student population using direct measures. That Sage Memorial Hospital School of Nursing admitted only Native Americans, Hispanics and a small number of Asian students suggests that all thirty-two cadet nurses there were Native American, Hispanic or Asian.

At Santa Monica's, the mission of the school was to serve all people, and its location amid public housing projects for African Americans and Mexican American communities in the middle of low-income South Phoenix contributed to this mission. Given the occasional reports that Santa Monica's accepted African American students that other Phoenix schools of nursing would not, we can deduce that there were a number of students of color at Santa Monica's. However, a photo collage of the second graduating class that appeared in a local Arizona newspaper failed to demonstrate this diversity. Also, one nurse who studied at Santa Monica's and whose oral history was recorded by Joyce Finch in the 1980s recalled that most students there were white.

When racial or ethnic data are not available, a Hispanic surname analysis can be a proxy indicator of the proportion of a group that is of Hispanic origin, so I conducted a Hispanic surname analysis of the 710 Arizona cadet nurse membership cards. Around 13 percent of all students in the five schools had Hispanic surnames. Around 33 percent of Sage Memorial's students had Hispanic surnames, and 23 percent of Saint Mary's students had Hispanic surnames. The proportion of Hispanic-surnamed cadet nurses in Phoenix's three schools of nursing was much lower.

The membership card data failed to prove without a doubt that the cadet nurse program attracted large numbers of young people from the sizable Mexican-heritage, African American, Asian-heritage or Native American communities within the state of Arizona. However, given the histories of these schools of nursing, one can extrapolate that at least 21.7 percent, or 178 of the 818 students, were either of Hispanic heritage or Native American or Asian because they were either students at Sage Memorial (where no white students were admitted) or had Hispanic surnames. The percentage could also be higher because those without a Hispanic surname might have been of Hispanic heritage nonetheless. What is more difficult to determine is the number of cadet nurses at schools of nursing in Phoenix or Tucson who might have been African American or Asian.

Training Experiences of Cadet Nurses Who Arrived in Arizona After World War II

Joyce Finch, a professor in the School of Nursing at Arizona State University (ASU), collected the oral histories of twenty-five cadet nurses living in Arizona after World War II.[40] These nurses' stories included their recollections about their experiences in nursing school, including the senior cadet period at the end of their training.

These nurses came primarily from the Upper Midwest of the United States. As over half of the participating schools of nursing were in the Upper Midwest and the Northeast,[41] this pattern is not surprising. One of the cadets received her training in California, and one trained in Arizona.

Forty percent of the nurses interviewed graduated from nursing school in 1947 with the remaining 60 percent roughly evenly distributed across the duration of the program, from 1944 to 1948. Nurses who graduated before 1946 started nursing school before the U.S. Cadet Nurse Corps began operation. The corps continued operation after the war ended so that student nurses already in the pipeline could complete their program of study. They were not required to commit to any service requirements because the war had already ended before they graduated.

The majority of the nurses interviewed by Joyce Finch reported training in a hospital school of nursing, and two of the nurses received training in a university setting. One attended Stanford University and the second attended Syracuse University. The 25 nurses reported working and studying in hospitals outside Arizona that ranged in size from fewer than 100 beds to over 2,000. The average number of beds in the hospital setting of their schools of nursing was about 493. They reported classes ranging in size from as few as 18 students to as many as 125 with a graduation rate of as low as 49 percent to as high as 100 percent. Not all reported their schools having affiliations with other hospitals, but many reported affiliations with colleges and universities. Only 8 of the nurses reported affiliations with other hospitals; 21 of the nurses reported affiliations with colleges or universities. In general, hospital affiliations provided specialized training in areas not necessarily available at the student's school of nursing, such as special training in psychiatric or pediatric nursing. Through university affiliations, students received academic coursework in health-related sciences, such as chemistry, not generally available in a hospital setting.

HOW THE U.S. CADET NURSE CORPS MADE A DIFFERENCE

Federal funding made an enormous difference to young women in realizing their educational dreams by making this educational opportunity accessible. They grew up during the Great Depression, and few would have been able to afford the costs of going to nursing school. The comments of the twenty-five nurses who were interviewed by Joyce Finch in the 1980s reflected this reality. Seventeen nurses stated explicitly that were it not for the funding, they probably would not have been able to go to nursing school. In some cases, the financial support influenced a decision to enter nursing, a direction that they might not have taken without the financial incentive. In other cases, the financial support was appreciated because it took the burden off their families, who were still recovering from the effects of the Great Depression. This sentiment pervaded their comments:

> *As far as finances were concerned, it certainly made a big difference. I think the stipend at the time was $15 per month, which enabled us to take care of our own personal needs. We didn't have to go home and call on our parents for that. Most of our parents were not really too well off at that time...I had planned to be a nurse from the time I can remember. In fact, I think I borrowed the money to go into the school. It was like $87 or something like that, and I borrowed the money from a brother of mine. But, I would have made it through no matter what, but* [the Cadet Corps] *just made it a lot easier.*
>
> —*Lucile Flores*

> *We were very poor people...I would not have been a nurse had it not been for them. I had no way, my parents were from Ireland, they were very poor; they had lost the resources they had accumulated in '29 and my father never really recovered from that.*
>
> —*Margaret Clements*

> *I think eventually I would have, as I was saving my money, but very slowly. One didn't make much money at that time. I was getting ready to look into loans for Meadville Hospital, Meadville, PA. I also had checked two other training schools when this opportunity presented itself* [the Cadet Nurse Corps], *which solved my problem, as well as for many others. I had begun to think that I would never get the money saved, as money was not easy to*

come by…I would have been unable to go into nurse' training, if it had not been for the Cadet Nurse Corps.

—Katherine Day

I would have had to wait another year, or maybe more. I did have enough money for tuition saved up, but you know, our wages were low. I came out of high school and I didn't have any money; well, I had had some college but I was doing that part time too.

—Eugenia Dormady

My mother could not have afforded to send me away to school. I would have probably ended up behind a drugstore counter, or [in] *a five and dime store.*

—Ruby Gordon

I would not have been a nurse if it weren't for that because we did not have the funds. My folks didn't have the money to send us.

—Bernice Green

I know that at the time that the opportunity for enrolling or whatever it was in the Cadet Program came around, that it was pretty much of a God-send for me, because financially I was very strapped. My family could not provide me with anything more than just the monthly package of goodies that they would send, but they were not able to provide any financial support.

—Rosemary Johnson

At the point that I found out about this opportunity I wanted both a college education and a nursing education. My parents couldn't afford for me to have both. I don't know what I would have chosen, I really don't. I might not have gone through with nursing.

—Elaine Katzman

For one thing I didn't need to borrow the money—I was going to borrow it from my parents.

—Frances Knudson

I wasn't planning to be a nurse. In fact, I wanted to be a nutritionist and had all my papers in to Cornell University. I heard about the Cadet Corps, I guess I just read about it or something, and I decided that that was a pretty good deal. My mother decided that it was an excellent deal since she really didn't have too much money. She really thought that was wonderful and that I definitely should try it. So when I began to make inquiry about it and found out that financially it would be a great relief for my mom, I just decided to sign up.

—Georgia Macdonough

It would have been harder because my parents didn't have all that much money.

—June Niccum

It certainly took away any financial worries, as I recall.

—Elaine Sabel

[My parents couldn't]...*afford it, although my sister did go into nurses' training, well she had to pay her own way. But it was hard on her and my parents, so I was glad that I was able to have Uncle Sam pick up the tab.*

—Jane Yettke

However, it was not only financial motivations that prompted these women to become cadet nurses. The program offered young women the opportunity to serve their country. They had the opportunity to become part of a bigger world than the one in which they grew up. It opened them up to consider personal and professional directions that they might not have considered without it. It was a transformative experience. Comments illustrative of this sentiment include these examples:

It just sounded like a great opportunity and I would have no qualms about going into the service after my training. I thought the service was great. I was raised that way. My Dad was so patriotic, and he instilled that in all of us. I mean, to fight for your country was just wonderful.

—Constance Besch

The experience made it very sure in my mind that I was going into public health, and it never varied—for 41 years I have not changed my mind.

—Joan Douglas

Well, I think the Cadet Nurse Corps made the difference of sort of making you feel a part of what was going on at the time. Making you feel that if you were needed you'd be able to go, and that there was more or less of an equality between the men being needed and the female being needed.

—Clara Gilmore

See, had it not been for the Second World War and the funding of the Bolton Act, I may never have been able to get my initial start. And I think that that's where I got it. I think that I grew, personally, and obviously, professionally. And educationally and in any other kind of way, I grew from that little beginning. That was my opportunity. I took it, not realizing at that time...And as I look back, and I have thought of this many times over, how appreciative I am to the U.S. Government. To this day, I do not mind paying whatever taxes they say I owe. It does not even bother me, because I feel that that was my movement from high school to a career that has been really very rewarding to me. Even though at one point, I wanted to hop out of it and did so for a year, I came right back.

—Ruby Gordon

You felt like you were part of the group. There was much more of a group sense and a nationalistic type of sense, too, because of the War at the time and relatives being away in the service. It made you feel like you were doing your bit. I fully intended to go into the service, but it just happened the War was over before I graduated, so I did not have to fulfill that commitment.

—Elaine Katzman

It brought me away from, a little bit at least, away from the sheltered life that I had had. At college I attended a church college, also a church affiliated hospital. We were quite sheltered. I was one, of course, to abide by the rules and I feel that it was good for me to get out and meet a different type of people, to learn to really realize and know a few different types of people.

—Shirley Kirking

It really extended my education. I saw so many more things than I would have in my home school—the different injuries and that sort of thing. I made a lot of friends.

—Doris Meharry

Senior Cadet Experience

An innovative feature of the program was a six-month-long supervised clinical experience during the last six months of their program of study that provided for students to engage in federal service in such settings as veterans administration, Indian Service or military hospitals, as well as in civilian hospitals. This feature of the program was made available unevenly. In some cases, student nurses were not apprised of this opportunity because the hospital where they were being trained was in such great need for nurses that they were not permitted to leave. Among the twenty-five cadet nurses interviewed by Joyce Finch, eight reported that they stayed in their home school of nursing during the last six months, and they assumed greater responsibility during this time. The rest of the group reported service in other settings, such as Bureau of Indian Affairs reservation hospitals, military hospitals, VA hospitals, rural nursing and civilian hospitals other than their home hospital.

Ruby Gordon was a student at Santa Monica's Hospital in Phoenix, where no one left the city for the last six months, but she said:

> *We did have options of how we wanted to spend our last six months in clinical experiences. I chose mine in Emergency Room. There were several of the students who worked with the then Phoenix Health Department…But at any rate, perhaps half a dozen of my classmates were allowed that option to serve in public health. I didn't choose it myself. But other than that, we had no other kinds of affiliations.*

This was apparently not an uncommon practice, as a number of the nurses reported similarly that they were not permitted to leave their home hospital because they were needed there. A few students from a class might have applied and been selected for a senior experience elsewhere; some might have been offered the opportunity but opted to stay in their home hospital. Those who stayed might have gone to other local facilities during the last six months, in a setup similar to a senior experience, or the opportunity might not have been offered.

Lucile Flores reported no senior experience in another facility. She indicated that because the hospital was so short of nurses that they were unable to permit students to go elsewhere for the last six months. Instead, she

> *worked with the head* [nurses]. *Well they were called supervisors then. Now they would be either head nurse or coordinator, and I was more or less working under her. By May, before I graduated, the supervisor became very ill, and I more or less stepped in. By the time I graduated, I filled her position. At the time that was supervision. I worked in that position for a year before I left.*

Charlotte Katona and June Niccum had senior experiences in VA hospitals. Charlotte had clinical experiences in all services—medical, surgical and chronic care. There was an educational coordinator at the VA hospital who oversaw the objectives for their learning or practice experiences. Charlotte reported that they presented papers and were on duty at least forty hours per week. They were supervised by a charge nurse or head nurse and did case-method nursing and some team nursing. June Niccum was one of only two students in her class who opted to go away for a senior experience, for which she specialized in orthopedics, quadriplegia and tuberculosis. Though there were not many classes, she was supervised by head nurses on the floor at the VA hospital where she served.

A number of the nurses interviewed by Joyce Finch had their senior experiences in civilian settings. Elaine Katzman selected obstetrics for her senior experience specialization and went to the Cornell Medical Center, where, in addition to supervised patient care, she participated in seminars. Shirley Kirking opted for rural nursing in Grand Rapids, Minnesota, where she worked in the hospital there and also explored industrial nursing in a paper mill, an area in which she was interested but which she never entered. Georgia Macdonough opted to stay in her home hospital because it gave her an opportunity to learn how to be an administrator. During the last six months, she became an acting head nurse, which put her in a good position to learn some management skills that she probably would never have had, had she gone away.

In Rosemary Johnson's case, the war ended before she was ready to serve at the San Diego Naval Base. She changed her plans and took her last six months in mental health and psychiatric nursing at a psychiatric hospital.

Those who took advantage of the senior experience reported in general that it was a most valuable opportunity. For example, Joan Douglas, a cadet nurse at Stanford University, spent her last six months of training at a Bureau of Indian Affairs hospital in Fort Defiance, Arizona. She was about forty miles away from Ganado, Arizona, and the Sage Memorial Hospital. She noted:

> *So, I came to Fort Defiance, Arizona, at Window Rock, and that was my first experience away from Stanford. It was an experience you couldn't buy any place in the world, outside of India...It was a good thing—I knew what to do because I was a five-year person. I had had every kind of experience at Stanford. I'd been Charge Nurse, I'd been a Night Supervisor, I knew how to do the report. I was a great Surgical Nurse at that time and*

> *I can remember setting up for surgeries there at the hospital in Window Rock at Fort Defiance and doing all those things. But I knew how to do it because I'd done more than I ever needed to do as a student. During the War we had to do many things.*

Joan also reported that the experience on the Indian Reservation solidified her commitment to public health nursing.

REFLECTIONS AT THE END OF THEIR CAREERS

Joyce Finch's oral history collection also included the stories of these twenty-five cadet nurses' experiences after World War II to 1987, when they would have been approaching the end of their careers or had already retired. Their stories included recollections of their career trajectories, family lives, roles in the feminist movement and other reflections over their life experiences and the nursing profession after World War II. Almost half of these nurses arrived in Arizona earlier in their careers in the period before the 1970s. This group would have been between their early twenties and late forties when they arrived in Arizona. Those who arrived in the 1970s or 1980s would have been in their fifties or sixties.

Balancing Career, Education, and Family After the War

Their stories revealed at least 180 unique employers over the course of their collective careers. All of the twenty-five nurses served as staff nurses in hospitals, and some began their careers as nurses in the hospital where they received their training. However, each had a different set of circumstances that led her to balance career, family and educational advancement differently. For some, the balance favored home and family; for others, the balance favored workplace responsibilities, and for the third group, the balance favored scholarship and education for future generations of nurses. Among this last group of women were professors of nursing at Arizona State University; nursing home administrators; staff or supervising nurses in civilian, military and veterans administration hospitals; doctor's office nurse; public health and community health nurses; and nurses in emerging specializations, such as nurse practitioner, school nurse practitioner, emergency room nurse and Indian Service nurse.

Throughout their careers, they took advantage of continuing education opportunities offered by employers or professional organizations to advance their skills and to learn new ones for emerging fields within nursing, such as school nursing, geriatric nursing and nurse practitioner. Ten of the twenty-five pursued higher education and earned a baccalaureate, generally a bachelor of science in nursing. Five went on to pursue a master's degree in nursing, counseling or education; one earned a graduate certificate in public health, and four earned a doctorate in nursing or education. Some alternated between full-time study at college and work, and others were somehow able to study full time while working part time as nurses, combined work with education for financial or other reasons or took leaves of absence or sabbaticals.

How each of these twenty-five nurses balanced the demands of career, continuing education and family responsibilities varied, but in general, each nurse's trajectory trended more heavily in one of three patterns over the other two. I call these patterns career practitioner, hands-on nursing and nursing and public health education leader. The career practitioner's trajectory reflected, in general, a continuous series of nursing positions in hospital or related settings, usually accompanied by progressively increasing levels of management responsibility. The hands-on nurse tucked her nursing career in between family responsibilities, and the series of nursing positions held was interrupted and less likely to reflect progressively increasing levels of responsibility. The nursing and public health education leader held a continuous series of positions with increasing responsibility, which also required creativity and leadership skills.

The career practitioner orientation predominated in five nurses' stories. They spent the majority of their careers in hospital-based nursing positions with progressively increasing levels of responsibility. In some cases, they took the initiative to address procedural issues and improve nursing practice in their work settings. Though they were all married and had children, their stories reflected marriages that appeared to allow for the needs or desires of both spouses to work and for both spouses and their children to contribute to the household operation in Arizona. For instance, in one case, one spouse worked days, and the other nights, so that they could share the one car they owned to get to and from work. In another case, both arranged work schedules so that they could sleep while children were at school or cared for by their grandparents.

Hands-on nursing dominated the careers of twelve nurses. These women held a series of positions in a number of places around the country, or they participated in some sort of entrepreneurial activity with their husbands. Their mobility was because of their investment in their husbands' work or a child's or other relative's health. Their stories did not describe career trajectories reflective of strategically planned progressively increasing levels of responsibility in nursing outside the home. For at least some of this group, they spoke of husbands who did not want them to work outside the home, a stance that sometimes changed over time.

In eight nurses' stories, a nursing and public health education leader pattern predominated. One was involved in the development of the nursing program in Glendale Community College of the Maricopa County Community College System. Another led in the development of school nursing and school nurse practitioner roles and encouraged a third to work on public health nursing and education with Native American tribes in northern Arizona. A fourth cadet nurse stood out as an instructor at the University of Arizona, and the remaining four nurses were instrumental in the development of undergraduate and graduate nursing programs at Arizona State University.

Changing Practice in Changing Times

To effect changes brought by the U.S. Cadet Nurse Corps required skilled leadership and innovative ideas not only about nursing practice but also about the role of women. Joyce Finch asked the nurses for their perspectives on their roles as leaders or innovators during their careers, as well as their perspectives on the Women's Movement and their participation in it.

LEADERSHIP

The nurses' stories reflected an array of perspectives on what leadership is, from its distinction from followership or management to leadership as a role. Most of the nurses saw themselves as leaders, but a number of them did not. Among those who did not see themselves as leaders, June Niccum acknowledged that others considered her a leader, and Leona Pearson had simply never considered it and had no answer. Surprisingly, Frances Knudsen, whose story about her career trajectory reflected leadership, did not think she was especially a leader. Marylou Gertz did not consider herself a leader in general nursing but felt she could have been a leader had she gone back for her bachelor's degree when ASU started its nursing program. However, she also stated that she wouldn't have been able to because of work. In the end, she decided forego her own education and devote herself to influencing her sons to achieve in school.

Among those who acknowledge that they were leaders, a number of stories reflected a leadership that is associated with equipping others so that they can succeed. Lucile Flores said:

> *Maybe you encouraged someone to go on to school. I can think of one person. That very first class that this person took (she now has her Master's). You can sit in a corner and get fulfillment from watching somebody else get the credit or go ahead, where you're still down here. But you're still guiding people here and there, and this is where I think that I feel I was a leader.*

And Constance Besch had this to say: "I love to teach them. I love to show them things, I like to show them how to do things."

Another nurse saw leadership as a responsibility to ensure that tasks that people are unable to do get done. According to Margaret Clements:

> *I haven't always chosen that* [being a leader]. *It's simply that you see a job to be done, it isn't that you are trying to assume any…If anything, I had always seen leadership primarily as a responsibility. You see something that's not being done, and there's no one else who can or will do it, so you do it. And you quickly summon all the necessary requisites forward. However you can, you do it.*

Barbara Miller viewed leadership as a role: "I think I've been a leader, just going back and thinking about all the things and some of the people that I encouraged to pursue higher levels [of education]. Also in the ANA, in which I have always been active, I had some leadership roles."

Jane Yettke saw leadership as communication of knowledge and new ideas:

> *Well, sometimes I probably say things I shouldn't. But, you know, someone says, "Why didn't you speak up" or something. Well, I'm the one that speaks up, I let people know my idea. So I don't know—maybe I'm a leader…Sometimes I think I'm a follower, and other times maybe I am a leader. It depends—if I know the subject matter and I'm real gung ho on something I guess I'm a leader.*

Margaret Clements recognized her leadership retrospectively in her professional practice:

> *Now that I've been to school, I recognize—when we studied modes of leadership and management, and so on, I sorta laughed and looked at myself and thought, "So that's what you were doing." I recognized then when I had to study it that I had recognized the differences in maturity levels of people and conducted myself according to that. I didn't have the training, but I recognized it when I was able to label it in school at University of Phoenix. It was a very interesting study, and of course, I learned all sorts of things in those courses. But that's when I said, "So, I'm a leader, how do you like that."*

INNOVATION

One of the nurses defined innovation as trying something new. With this definition in mind, the nurses' stories were sprinkled with tangible ways in which they considered themselves innovators:

For Margaret Clements, Rosemary Johnson and Donna Malone, innovation meant helping people succeed. Clements stated:

> *When I was a charge nurse, I came back into nursing and I acquired some different skills in real estate. I saw that the care was not what I thought it should be and I saw the need for training of the unskilled personnel at bedside. One of the first things I did there was to set it up so that I had nurses who were able and willing to work weekends so that I could offer five days a week, Monday through Friday to these nurses. And of course, they loved it and it worked. It worked. So I had no turnover to speak of, had excellent nurses. For nursing assistants I had different scheduling, but I tried to give them as much as possible, things that they needed, I tried to meet their needs. And then in turn, I expected them to meet the needs of the patients. Whatever changes were necessary, we did. But, of all those years being Director of Nursing and Administrator, and so on, that was the one thing that I demanded. And I demanded it of myself and of the staff—that they put the patient first. I really feel strongly about that. Everything had to be measured from whether it benefitted the patients or not. And they had to come first.*

Johnson recalled, "The phenomenon that I experienced [was] of being moved into positions where the innovator role could be developed that I never would have anticipated."

Malone said:

> *I have worked on some little procedures and trying to update them and make them simpler. Nothing that you would patent or anything like that, but just within my own working area. There are just little things. I think I was the first one in our hospital—it may not sound good on your tape—when you're putting in a Foley catheter to hook up your tubing first and then you don't have to worry about the urine getting all over when you're hooking up the tubing again. And they were amazed that I did that. Now they come with that type of system.*

Joyce Finch had no problem with Donna's example on tape because Donna was trying to improve the job and make it easier for herself and the patient. According to Joyce Finch, "That's innovation."

For Katherine Day, innovation meant changing practice to ensure the best outcomes for patients:

> *Well, I think in the past I did. But then, you know, you get the younger nurses and they don't want to listen and they don't want to try things. I remember one nurse got so upset with a patient because she wouldn't take her digitalis at 10:00 in the morning. I said, "What was the reason she gave?" She said, "Because she takes it at bedtime, and doctor said she could do it." Well, you know I had to get the doctor to write an order to say that the patient could take the digitalis at bedtime. And I said, "This is ridiculous. Why should we try to regulate what a patient's been doing for years, so that they don't miss taking their medication?" I wanted to try at that time, if you call this innovation, to make a survey of the patients to see when and how they took their pills. Did they take it at bedtime, or when did they take it? And then, when I would send the patients home and they were to take it every six hours, the doctor would say to me, "Now you go ahead and explain how you take it." I said, "Well, most patients go to bed at 10:30 at night, after the news, between 10:30 and 11:00, and the majority of the older patients are up to go to the bathroom about 6:00 in the morning. Why can't we make it 6:00, then at 12:00, then at 6:00 p.m. and at 10:30 at night. So what, we don't always get the pills given on time either, and besides you have a half-hour leeway." He thought that was nice. But, what I wanted to do so many times is check with patients. And I've always wanted to do a survey on diabetics and cardiac.*

For Joan Douglas, the one nurse among the twenty-five who was a senior cadet on a reservation in Arizona, innovation meant getting out of the way so that new ideas could be tested:

> *I think so because we always looked at different ways to do things—like community outreach workers, how nursing worked with them. We did a lot of demonstrating and when we would develop a program like family planning or child development center, we looked at new and different ways to meet the needs, and how to use ourselves a little bit differently. So I think we were innovative and I think I allowed that and encouraged it. The staff always had opportunities; I saw that they had opportunities. If they wanted to try something—that I encouraged, that was great.*

For Ruby Gordon, the one nurse among the twenty-five who trained in an Arizona school of nursing, innovation meant making an impact on nursing education:

> *Well, yes I think so. I think I have plunged ahead and certainly feel that I made some impact on nursing education. When I came into this job in Associate Degree nursing I actually had been encouraged at that particular time…By the way, I didn't mention this earlier, but I had taken some course work at ASU, some of their regular Baccalaureate level courses. I had taken the one with Public Health, it was a six semester hour course at that time…And one of the cases that I had was a blind girl who had been allowed to keep her baby. She'd had a baby out of wedlock and she had been allowed to keep her baby. I did some sort of innovative things in my visits with her, writing these process recordings out. I taught her how to bathe that baby, the safety precautions, etc. Anyway, Rosemary had encouraged me to write that up, which I did. It was published in the* AJN, *way back whenever that was. Also, when I was at Saint Joseph's, someone had said nurses are always getting their backs injured. It seemed to be a prominent thing that they kept repeating over and over. So, one day I said to myself, "It just seems like we don't have that many injured backs." So I undertook to do a survey. They had not had a safety program at Saint Joseph's at that particular time. As a matter of fact, a lot of hospitals didn't have one. So, I did a survey. I took all of the occupational reports of injuries on the job. Actually, this was somewhere in the middle* ['60s], *as I recall. For the previous calendar year, I took all those reports and categorized the area of the body that was injured and all that kind of stuff. So, it was an after-the-fact type of survey.*

> *Actually, this was before I'd had a lot of course work in research methods. But at any rate, I had this big report. I thought I might as well send it off to* Hospitals, *you know, the* Journal of the American Hospital Association. *So, immediately they wanted it to publish it.*

For Elaine Katzman, Rosemary Johnson and Georgia Macdonough, innovation meant assuming new roles in nursing. Elaine Katzman reported living in many places and that the nurse practitioner role that emerged during her career was an unprecedented one. Where she saw a need for her colleagues to learn a new technique, she worked with them in instituting programs to fill that need. Rosemary Johnson's version of innovation was being moved into positions where she would develop as a thought leader. Innovation, in her experience, was not something planned; it just happened. Georgia Macdonough confessed that while in her career she would not have considered herself an innovator, but in hindsight, she noted, "Something must have been there because I kept getting these jobs that I didn't go after." Someone saw something in her.

In Georgia's case, Joyce Finch clearly saw her work in the school nurse practitioner role and setting up physical assessments in rural areas as innovative. What Georgia introduced might not have been planned to be groundbreaking, but in retrospect it was. Georgia was an innovative leader.

Finally, Eugenia Dormady considered herself avant-garde but never gave it much thought: "I suppose I am to some degree because I had to be innovative. Just raising a family you have to be innovative. If you [aren't], you're foundering, right? I think that I can take charge if I have to and be innovative, but I never thought of myself as that. I never gave it that much thought."

FEMINISM

The twenty-five nurses' stories reflected a number of perspectives on the women's movement, which was underway during their careers.

Eugenia Dormady acknowledged a change in social expectations for women that opened the door to their being homemakers and having careers. She was aware that change was in the air, but she felt fine about it. She thought perhaps that she was a women's liberator because her mother had been a very strong person who might have been working for women's rights had she not been born during the Victorian age. Eugenia noted, "I suppose nothing angers me more than to see women who are not given the recognition they should be given just because they are women." She had six daughters and three sons and claimed that the girls were inclined to be a bit scrappy because they learned it from her. Her advice to her daughters: "All of you have got to go to college, you've got to have something. No matter what. Just because you get married, you never know what's going to happen and you might need this. You've got to be educated."

Eugenia's mother thought the same. She pushed for her children to be educated, although Eugenia was in the first generation of her family to be born in the United States.

Joan Douglas spoke to the ways in which women worked together to lift one another up and to be inclusive. Her women's movement was one where women worked together to develop leadership and bring opportunities to women in communities where such opportunities might not exist. Joan spoke of listening and helping women do things they did not know they could do. As a community organizer, she reported doing a lot to develop that type of leadership. She also noted that the work was particularly challenging in rural areas for both men and women. She was instrumental in creating jobs through another federally funded program, the Comprehensive Education and Training Act (CETA),[42] for women seeking employment during the 1970s and whom other organizations would not accept. Joan recalled:

> *Interesting thing—when we were developing the course and describing how we were going to use community outreach workers, we needed to reach the people that needed to be reached. Our public health nurses were sometimes handicapped. We needed a young man with a beard and a guitar. We needed a young woman who had been* [on] *drugs at some time or other, or was a single parent. We needed a black woman. We needed a gypsy woman. We actually advertised, selected, recruited and trained—and you know, we ended up with five or six of them who had never* [worked]*; they went on to great jobs or they stayed with us for seven or eight or ten years, and did unique things, and went back to school and worked at the same time. So, it was fascinating. Nobody had ever cared or worked with them before, actually. And they made all the difference in the world. We changed the color and everything of our clinics, or our programs and so on, because we could really bring the people* [in]*—now we could communicate with them. So yes, that was pretty exciting. I think that was kind of helping the*

> *Women's Movement, because they later went on and did things—they held positions in the communities, and so on.*

Charlotte Katona did not see herself particularly involved in the women's movement, possibly because she did not feel the limitations that many women around her did. The way her family operated and raised her, as well as the type of man her husband was, did not impose limitations on her because of her gender. She was not anti–women's movement, but she did believe that opportunities offered depend a lot on the individual's abilities and preparation for them.

Shirley Kirking saw herself as part of the women's movement because she probably would have gone to work, even if necessity had not forced her to work.

Chapter 5

SELECTED ARIZONA CADET NURSE PROFILES

I became acquainted with many Arizona cadet nurses through their membership cards, interview transcripts and the generosity of their family and friends. All assuredly led remarkable lives. In this chapter, I will profile ten of them. Two trained in Arizona, and two were Latina. Two grew up in Arizona, and one of these two was born in Arizona. Those who trained elsewhere arrived in Arizona at different points in their adult lives, as early as immediately after World War II to as late as the early 1970s—early enough to have made their mark on nursing practice in postwar Arizona and, for some, also nationally and globally. These ten women's profiles are in chronological order. Sylvia Jiménez Almeyda was born in Arizona, and Jane Yettke arrived last, in 1979.

SYLVIA JIMÉNEZ ALMEYDA

Sylvia Jiménez Almeyda was born on November 3, 1917, in Clifton, Arizona, a copper mining camp in Greenlee County.[43] Shortly thereafter, Sylvia and her parents, Antonio and Josefa Gonzales Jiménez, moved to Miami, Arizona, where her father found laborer's work at the Miami Copper Company. After graduation in 1935 from Miami High School, Sylvia found work at a mine hospital in Miami, where she fixed salads for the patients, among other responsibilities. Over time, Sylvia became a secretary for Nurse

Catherine Beagin, who had helped her find her job at the hospital. Nurse Beagin also saw a career opportunity for Sylvia through the U.S. Cadet Nurse Corps.

The prospect of becoming a nurse was met with disapproval from her mother, who thought it undignified for a young woman to touch men. "Women were supposed to be at home, wash dishes and have babies," Sylvia said.[44] So Nurse Beagin put Sylvia in a car and brought her to Saint Mary's in Tucson.

In 1943, she became a member of the U.S. Cadet Nurse Corp. Within this program, Sylvia enrolled in Saint Mary's School of Nursing and began taking nurses' training in Tucson, graduating from Saint Mary's in 1945. Sylvia once said about her classmates at Saint Mary's, "The girls were from all over, Jews, not all Catholics—I got to understand people of different faiths. When you're a nurse, you have to work with different people."[45]

By then, her soldier husband-to-be, Alfred Almeyda, returned from his military service overseas to his home in Miami. He and Sylvia soon married and began their life together in California, where they lived until 1986. As a registered nurse, Sylvia established an exemplary record of service in major hospitals in California with a specialty in maternity and infant care. Sylvia retired after forty-five years in nursing. She and Alfred Almeyda returned to Miami, Arizona, in 1986 to enjoy a new life in retirement. The couple became active in community service work for the Our Lady of the Blessed Sacrament Catholic Church, the Miami Senior Center and the Bullion Plaza Cultural Center and Museum.

Of the 2010 enactment of SB 1070, Arizona's anti-illegal immigration legislation, which has been said to unfairly target Latinos, Sylvia says about her family, "We are U.S. citizens. We love our country. We served."[46]

JOAN DOUGLAS

Joan Douglas began her career in nursing in Arizona during her senior cadet experience through Stanford University at Fort Defiance in Window Rock, an experience that she reported strengthened her commitment to pursue public health as a career. Joan returned to Arizona in 1980 with her master's degree in public health, earned in 1959 at the University of North Carolina, and a wealth of experience in public health nursing and nurse education in the Pacific Northwest and northern California. Her first position in Arizona was teaching community health nursing at the ASU College of Nursing. Joan left that position in 1983 to join the Arizona State Health Department as a consultant on long-term care. From there, she went to work with the Office of Local Health Service under Georgia Macdonough. Her special assignment was with the Indian tribes on health issues. Joan did general consultation and staff education. She worked as part of an interdisciplinary team to help a tribe write a preventive health block grant to develop a program with a nutritionist, a nurse and a community nutrition worker for high cholesterol prevention in the community. She also spent a week with the Navajo and the Hopi tribes and some of the local health departments doing workshops on school health, Board of Nursing law and regulations and helping community health nurses and school nurses to use one another as resources.

Joan confessed that she didn't want to stay in nursing because she always wanted to be in public health. At the time when she went for her master's in public health, she also looked into being a veterinarian, but she reported that she could not connect public health with veterinary medicine.

Ruby Gordon

Ruby Gordon was the only cadet nurse whom Joyce Finch interviewed who also trained in Arizona, at Santa Monica's School of Nursing in Phoenix. Though she was not born in Arizona, her family came to Prescott, Arizona, in the mid-'40s from the South because her sister was asthmatic.

She became a single mother and, during the '50s, worked a series of jobs in the healthcare industry, including a position at a health insurance company, manager in a medical practice and a hospital staff nurse. Ruby worked her way through ASU, where she earned her bachelor's degree. In the late '50s, she continued in a master's program in counseling through the ASU College of Education (a nursing program did not yet exist at ASU or in Arizona at the time).

From there, Ruby went on to teach biology in the Phoenix Union High School district and subsequently moved on to the Glendale School District to teach biology there. She found that high school teaching was not for her and moved on to teach in the Saint Joseph's Hospital School of Nursing in Phoenix. At Saint Joseph's, Ruby also wrote a grant with a colleague that established a Coronary Care Unit in the hospital.

When Saint Joseph's closed the school of nursing, Ruby moved to Glendale Community College, where a nursing program for the western Maricopa County area was being established. Ruby represented the college at the Western Interstate Commission on Higher Education (WICHE), which was starting a five-year curriculum project in nursing at that time. That association helped Ruby develop the curriculum at Glendale Community College, where Ruby became the chairman for the Department of Nursing. After she completed the PhD in adult education and administration at Arizona State University, Ruby transferred to Phoenix College to teach nursing there, but she ended up teaching in an area with which she was not familiar. As with all the other challenging opportunities that she encountered in her career, Ruby sought out traineeships and funding for them to equip her for a new role.

When asked if she was satisfied with the decision to return to nursing, Ruby responded:

> *Oh, yes. I look back over all of my life. I guess I'm at a time in life when I look back, as some people do. There is hardly anything that I have done that I would not repeat again. I feel real pleased with the accomplishments that I've made. I've had a lot of people who have assisted me and fostered me, and listened to me through the years. I feel real comfortable. In fact, I can't think of anything that I have done or the way in which my career has gone that I would change. I feel very career-oriented, probably due to the circumstances of having been left by myself to raise a child. I frequently chuckle to myself that I probably got hung-up on education. But, I just had some kind of zest. To this day, I have a zest effect. I applied this past spring and participated in a pilot project the District had for VISIONS. It's like re-careering, and we each had to do something of interest. I got interested in Gerontology. In fact, I applied to ASU under the College of Public Programs. Naturally, they accepted me. They've got a lot of openings in this field.*

Ruby Gordon was one of the first two faculty members of nursing when Glendale Community College launched its nursing program in 1965. In 2009, she was recognized with a Special Award for Excellence for a career that spanned more than fifty years in nursing, health education and student counseling.

Ellamae Branstetter

Ellie Branstetter arrived in Arizona in 1945 after having been a head nurse in the hospital where she trained to be a nurse. She worked in Tucson as an emergency room nurse at Pima County Hospital for about six months.

After a short return to her home state of Missouri, Ellie returned to Arizona and worked at Santa Monica's Hospital in Phoenix as a supervisor and clinical instructor in their school of nursing. She had a year's college before she started nursing school. After a year at Santa Monica's, she went to the Indian Hospital in Phoenix as a staff nurse.

Ellie alternated work with the Visiting Nurse Service in Phoenix with study in Missouri and finished her undergraduate degree in public health at St. Louis University. Ellie returned to Arizona as a field instructor with the Visiting Nurse Service and became assistant director. Then she went off to the University of Minnesota to earn a master's in public health in mental health nursing. Her motivation to pursue the master's was her interest in teaching.

Ellie returned to Arizona in 1957 to address the lack of collegiate-based nursing programs in Arizona by helping to start the baccalaureate program in nursing at Arizona State University. As the nursing program grew from a department in the liberal arts college to an independent school within ASU, Ellie became assistant director of the school. A few years later, in 1962, she went to Chicago for her doctoral degree, which she completed in 1969. During her doctoral study, Ellie consulted with ASU on the development of their master's program in nursing. At the time, she was the only faculty member in the school with doctorate-level training. She served also as assistant dean, as well as chair of the graduate program, and taught an array of courses in her role as a faculty member in the school.

Ellie always wanted to stay in nursing "because I've changed jobs from time to time…I think if I'd been doing the same job, I would not have. But that's the nice thing about nursing—we can change roles."

Lucile Flores

Lucile Flores arrived in Arizona from Hutchinson, Kansas, directly after completing her training. She worked at Pima County Hospital and Tucson Medical Center Hospital and resided in both places in hospital-provided housing, which included meals and laundry services. She was a staff nurse in obstetrics.

In 1948, Lucile applied for admission to then Arizona State College (now known as Arizona State University) upon the urging of a friend who was a medical student at Pima County and her father. During this time, she also married. Lucile's husband returned to Kansas to finish his education at a community college.

Lucile started at Arizona State College as a full-time student living in the dorm and worked at Mesa Southside Hospital (now Desert Samaritan Hospital) on Saturdays and Sundays. She finished her degree in 1949 and went on to work at Good Samaritan Hospital as a pediatric supervisor and also taught pediatrics for one year. Lucile worked until the birth of her first child in 1951 and then returned to work in early 1952 as an evening supervisor for the hospital.

Lucile also took extension courses, taught by ASU professors and paid for by the hospital. In 1972, she went to work in geriatric nursing and took a course in gerontological nursing to prepare herself for her new role. From there, Lucile decided to move to California to work in a convalescent hospital as a geriatric nurse and, subsequently, a community hospital as an evening supervisor. Her family stayed behind in Arizona. Lucile returned to Arizona in 1973 and returned to work in a VA hospital as a staff nurse. This position was her last position before retirement.

Lucile always wanted to stay in nursing because she and her family thought they needed the money, but it was primarily for self-satisfaction. It was something she had always wanted to do, and she did it.

BERNICE GREEN

Bernice Green arrived in Arizona in 1955. She was a U.S. Public Health Service nurse with the Bureau of Indian Affairs who transferred from the Indian Reservation in Rosebud, South Dakota, to the Phoenix Indian Medical Center. The nursing supervisor at Rosebud had been transferred to Phoenix and was having trouble keeping nurses because if they were given a shift they didn't want, they'd just quit. There were many nursing positions available in the Phoenix area. So her plan was to pull in a few career nurses to stabilize the staff. Bernice was one of those career nurses. In 1962, Bernice retired. Her husband was trying to finish at the university, and she had two children at home: "In those days there weren't daycare centers. It was very difficult to find somebody who could understand my rotating shift, my rotating days off and on call. One of my girls had had 12 babysitters, and the other one 14. They were two and four years old. It was very traumatic for them, for me, and for the whole family."

Bernice was also concerned about the quality of care at the Indian Medical Center:

> *Patients would be brought from the Reservation and they would be, supposedly, admitted to be worked up. Some of them would sit there for three and four months without being worked up. I got the impression at the time if they didn't keep the beds full, then they'd lose some funds. This was very traumatic, because these people had farms, they had families. It really hurt to see that happen, and I had not found any way to do anything about it.*

She retired to full-time parenting and community service, including developing program resources—a girl's club and a daycare center—in an old neighborhood that was being redeveloped, until about 1971. Her daughters attended the Mitchell School, which also served that neighborhood.

Bernice returned to nursing as a public health nurse for the child health component at a Comprehensive Education and Training Act program site in South Phoenix. The parents and the children would be picked up at their homes by bus or other transportation and brought to the daycare, where the parents would leave the children and then go on to school or work. Bernice held a clinic in each daycare once a month. A doctor did physicals on those infants and children who were new to the program. A nurse from the Headstart Program would come along to give immunizations. Bernice went to the two school centers where the parents were to interview newly enrolled students and get the medical history on their children. She taught the staff proper procedures for the care of children when they are sick and for sanitary food preparation. After about two and a half years, the program's funding ended, and Bernice transferred to her final position in a program in maternity, child health and family planning.

LEONA PEARSON

Leona Pearson graduated from nursing school in 1944 and worked a number of months in her home hospital in St. Joseph, Missouri. She served as an army nurse stationed at Fitzsimmons Hospital in Denver for about a year during World War II and decided that a career in the army was not for her. Leona quit nursing for a while after her three children were born and returned to part-time service shortly after her third child was born in 1956. She advanced to charge nurse and then became director of nursing at another hospital and worked there until arriving in Arizona in July 1961. Neither Leona nor her husband had jobs when they arrived. Leona "got restless" and decided she had to work, and by October, both had jobs. They shared the one car they owned: he worked during the day, and she worked nights at Good Samaritan Hospital in Phoenix. Leona worked in the Medical-Surgical Department for one year and then in intensive care on the night shift for a couple years. Then Leona applied for and got the assistant head nurse job on an orthopedic floor, followed by an assistant head nurse position in the intensive care unit, where she worked for a couple years. Finally, Leona moved to a supervisor position for the afternoon shift, where she worked for about a year. In 1962, Leona began taking classes in nursing at ASU. Some courses were offered at the hospital and some on campus at ASU. In 1967, the director of the infirmary at ASU invited Leona to work there. She worked there for about a year and a half because it reduced the commute to work and made it easier for her to study, but Leona found this kind of nursing boring. During the summer, when the infirmary was closed, Leona worked at Camelback Hospital, returned to the ASU infirmary in the fall and moved on to the Scottsdale Memorial Hospital. At Scottsdale Memorial Hospital, she worked in the recovery room and, while learning this new area, worked to improve recovery room practice.

> *When I went there* [Scottsdale Memorial] *I set up a program for pre- and post-op teaching. Kay Lewis from Good Samaritan was one of the pioneers in doing the pre- and post-op teaching. I knew her when I was working there. I dug out her* AJN [*American Journal of Nursing*] *articles. They helped me an awful lot. Well, they were thinking about doing it before I started working there, but the way they did it... They didn't spend the time that they needed to spend. They didn't cover the things that Kay had in her article. I don't know if they read it or not, but I felt that it needed to be revised and perfected. Working the 3 to 11 shift, the people on 3 to 11*

were the ones who did the pre- and post-op teaching. So, I set up some better guidelines for that.

In 1976, Leona moved to the Outpatient Surgery Center of Scottsdale Memorial, a hospital-affiliated center, "the first one of that kind in the whole world." She coordinated the post-operative area. Joyce Finch noted that it sounded like a lot of what Leona suggested came to pass or got into the guidelines instructions. Leona agreed.

At the time of the interview in 1987, Leona reported that she was taking a course in research for general professional development, but "in the back of my mind I would like to do a research project of some kind and do some writing of some kind. I have a lot of information and a lot of ideas, but I'll probably take another course in creative writing or something like that before I stop all this business."

She reached the point in her program of study at ASU when she would have to study full time; she could not do that because she had to work. In 1984, Leona finished the BSN at the University of Phoenix, which had just opened its BSN program. She calculated that it was less expensive at the University of Phoenix than at ASU because she did not have to stop working.

Leona liked nursing as a career: "I never actually left nursing to do anything. I thought about it in my own mind, but I like the service, and never wanted to leave it."

Clara Gilmore

When Clara Gilmore arrived in Arizona in 1961, she went to work almost immediately at the Valley View Hospital in Phoenix. It was a small, general hospital in what at the time was the edge of town. Clara worked there full time for about three months and had to leave because of childcare issues when her husband was out of town a lot for his job. Clara worked in the infirmary at Grand Canyon University for twenty-five years. She also earned her bachelor's degree in education with a minor in health at Grand Canyon in 1973, which was her best option, given the difficulties associated with traveling to ASU for a nursing program and having young children at home. Despite having two daughters at home and a husband who was frequently out of town for his construction business, Clara always worked, keeping in mind the need to weave her work around her family responsibilities:

> *After we moved out here my husband, who is since retired, he was in construction and he worked with the big powerhouses all over the state. So, many times he would be gone and the girls and I would be home. And yet, the only time I had problems was when I was trying to work at the hospital, and that schedule did not work with mine. Then when I started down here* [at Grand Canyon University], *I started out only part-time, four hours a day with the weekends off. Of course, I was on call 24 hours a day. But, the hours there corresponded to the hours that our girls were at school. Gradually as they became older I became more involved in work and was able to work longer. So it worked out very well, really.*

Clara worked because she wanted to. She felt she had something to contribute. She was confident that she could have worked any place in town and would have been financially secure.

Georgia Macdonough

In 1963, Georgia Macdonough arrived in Arizona from Long Island, New York, where she had already earned a bachelor's degree and begun her career as a school nurse teacher. The relocation was because of her husband's job. Georgia started her career in school nursing in Arizona as the result of an informational interview that she had with a district superintendent. She introduced the teaching component into school nursing in Arizona that she learned in New York. Georgia earned a master's degree in counseling education from ASU because at the time there was no nursing program at ASU. She kept current with nursing through involvement with the Arizona Nurse's Association and summer work in hospitals as a staff nurse. Because of her experience with a type of school nursing that was not common practice in Arizona at the time, Georgia was recruited by the Arizona State Health Department to serve as school nurse consultant. As part of this work, she developed a course in school nursing at Phoenix College, a local community college. Georgia also expanded the scope of the course so that it could be an upper-division undergraduate course and taught it at ASU. The course was for not only new school nurses but also any school nurse who wanted to increase her capacity in the field. Georgia also worked in developing a community health specialty in the nursing program at ASU. She increased her capacity by going to Colorado to prepare to become a certified school nurse practitioner. With the support of her employer, Georgia was able to balance the demands of work with the demands of this program. From the position of school nurse consultant, Georgia went on to become director of local health, the liaison office between the county health departments and other health departments and the state. This office was also directed to take care of border health issues, to be responsible for rural health and to interface with Indian Health. Georgia spoke of a number of issues that her office was responsible for addressing:

> *Our office was, by statute, given the responsibility to chair the committee that looked at the status of nursing in Arizona and to make plans for the future. So that's the hot issue of the day in terms of nursing. In terms of state work with the counties, the issue is probably contracts—how this State Health Department can get the work in public health done in the counties by contracting so that the counties can get some money to do the job that needs to be done. We're really very much involved in those issues. In terms of Indian health, I think the big issue is the fact that we have to figure out how we can assist the tribes for members who live on the reservation, that need involuntary commitment to the psychiatric hospital, along with the issue of who pays. So we're boxed up in that because the State feels that Indian Health Service by statute has the responsibility to provide health care for the Indians on the reservation, be it physical or mental health. They think that the State ought to be providing in-patient care for all state citizens. So we're in the middle of that kind of thing. The Border Health issue, the big one is how do we get our American citizens who go over across the line for recreational purposes and get into either illness or accident situations evacuated from across the line so that they get good health intervention, good emergency care intervention, and that's what we're working on there.*

Georgia reported always being satisfied in nursing: "Especially for somebody who started out not even knowing that there was a career in nursing. I liked it once I got into it, and I never wanted to be anything else."

Jane Yettke

The bulk of Jane Yettke's career took place before her arrival in Arizona in 1979. She trained in Iowa and served as a staff or charge nurse in the air force (reaching the rank of major in the reserves), in military hospitals (Letterman Army Hospital, California; Scott Air Force Base, Illinois), in VA hospitals (Jefferson Barracks and John Cochran, St. Louis, Missouri) and in university teaching hospitals (Iowa City; Ann Arbor, Michigan). She also served in a university student health infirmary (Michigan) and was a summer camp nurse (Michigan).

Jane was an air force nurse during the Korean conflict and was called up from the reserves during the Pueblo incident. She also cared for soldiers returning from the battlefield during the war in Vietnam. During the police action in Korea, Jane was stationed at Kaiser Air Force Base in Mississippi. During the Pueblo incident in 1968, she was initially assigned to Hamilton Air Force Base in California and was transferred to Scott Air Force Base in Illinois.

At Kaiser, First Lieutenant Jane was a staff nurse in the ear, nose and throat ward and a charge nurse in the pediatrics ward until she was separated from the service in 1952. Jane also conducted training for medics. From Kaiser, on the urging of a friend, Jane went to University Hospital in Ann Arbor and a summer camp elsewhere in Michigan. In 1953, she went back to Iowa City and worked in orthopedics. At the urging of another girlfriend, Jane went to San Francisco to work at Letterman Army Hospital as a civilian nurse in the officers' ward. She had been there for fourteen years when her reserve unit was recalled during the Pueblo incident in 1968. Jane was assigned to Scott Air Force Base in Illinois and worked first in the RON (Remain Overnight) ward for patients arriving by Air Evac. Jane found working with patients she would know for only a few hours frustrating, so she requested and was given an assignment in the General Hospital. She was in charge of the medical ward.

Jane married in November 1969 and left active duty in January 1970. From there, she went to work in the VA hospitals in St. Louis. Jane started in John Cochran and subsequently transferred to Jefferson Barracks, her first choice. She worked with the long-term, chronically ill patients in a combination of charge and staff positions. During days, Jane was generally a staff nurse; during evenings and nights, as the only nurse, she was in charge. Jefferson Barracks was her last position before moving to Arizona.

In Mesa, Jane was a staff nurse at Desert Samaritan Hospital working part time in the evenings for six months. Then she worked at Williams Air Force Base in Mesa in a temporary Civil Service position that reverted to military at the end of a year. She was laid off from that position. Her last job was at the Los Flores Nursing Home. Jane navigated well the transition from hospital nursing to nursing home care and decided to retire in 1983.

Jane enjoyed being a nurse, but in the end, she decided that the time had come to end her career: "I used to love going to work when I was working at Letterman, but I guess maybe the type of people I was taking care of or else some of the young doctors…Maybe it was because I was getting older, maybe they thought I didn't know what I was saying or doing, I don't know. I just decided it was time to hang up my hat."

CONCLUSION

I have described the U.S. Cadet Nurse Corps program features and history and reviewed the context in which nursing students trained in Arizona's five participating nursing schools. I also explored complementary primary and secondary sources about U.S. Cadet Nurses in or of Arizona. When considered together, an impression about the Cadet Nurse Corps and cadet nurses emerges that prompts me to pose additional questions about the representativeness of this story for Arizona and in general. For instance, to what extent do the experiences of minority cadet nurses in Arizona represent the experiences of racial or ethnic minority cadet nurses nationally? To what extent was the opportunity to graduate, and therefore to be able to become a cadet nurse, equitably distributed in the Arizona educational system?

These two data sets are also augmented by other resources. I learned about the U.S. Cadet Nurse Corps from documenting the stories of other cadet nurses outside Arizona since 2011 through the participatory uscadetnurse.org website.[47] I have also reviewed oral history transcripts or recordings of other cadet nurses outside Arizona, read or listened to accounts of cadet nurse experiences authored by other cadet nurses and listened to cadet nurses' family members' recollections of their deceased mother's, aunt's or sibling's experiences as a cadet nurse.[48] I also grew up as the daughter of a cadet nurse, who trained in then rural Westchester County, New York.

Sometimes, I learned more about a cadet nurse trained in Arizona when I learned of her passing. Ana Marie Baez and Clara Rebecca Nourse were Arizona cadet nurses whom I learned about through their obituary notices.[49]

Ana Marie Baez came to the United States from Mexico City with her family while she was a child. She grew up in the U.S. Southwest and graduated from Menaul School in Albuquerque, New Mexico. She was one of the first Hispanic graduates at the Sage Memorial Hospital and worked as a nurse for sixty-six years. Clara Rebecca Nourse at first went to the University of Arizona to study library science. While there, she took a class in nursing and discovered her passion—taking care of people. She decided to become a nurse and trained at Santa Monica's Hospital in Phoenix.

Except possibly for Ruby Gordon, Clara Rebecca Nourse, Ana Marie Baez and Sylvia Jiménez, I know less about cadet nurses who trained in Arizona than I do about cadet nurses who came to Arizona after training elsewhere. I do not know as much about cadet nurses' training experiences in Arizona; their senior cadet experience; their lives after World War II; and their thoughts about leadership, innovation and the women's movement. I do not know how their stories might be similar to or different from the stories of the twenty-five nurses in Arizona who trained elsewhere. Listening to additional Arizona cadet nurses tell their stories would be an important step in bridging this gap. However, achieving this goal may be easier said than done: these women are at least eighty-eight years old and may not be available for one reason or another.

Conversely, the oral histories provided a window into the stories of twenty-five nurses who happened to be living in Arizona in 1987, when Joyce Finch interviewed them, but did not include details that their card file data would have provided. We know what their training experiences were like in nursing school and how they occupied themselves professionally, educationally and personally since World War II. However, the oral histories did not provide information about their fathers', guardians' or spouses' occupations.

These limitations notwithstanding, the oral histories and the few available additional stories about cadet nurses trained in Arizona provided a window into experiences at the cutting edge of the time during and after World War II. All of these women kept to the promise to serve as nurses in essential roles in civilian, military or Indian Service hospitals for the duration of the war. One served in the military during subsequent conflicts in the 1950s and 1960s. They experienced the miracles of modern medicine in fighting bacterial infections, tuberculosis and polio that were not available when people like Lulu Clifton arrived in Arizona decades before in search of a cure. They were at the forefront of new specialties in nursing: the school nurse teacher, school nurse practitioner, emergency room nurse and geriatric nurse. They were there for the introduction of new forms of nursing practice in life care facilities, nursing homes, long-term care facilities and hospital-affiliated outpatient surgery facilities. They experienced new organizational arrangements in hospitals as staff nurses, charge nurses, primary nurses, admitting nurses, head nurses, supervisors, directors of nursing and a number of other titles as hospitals grew over time. Some nurses drove change, and others simply endured it.

Through these complementary stories, a cohesive whole begins to take shape that sheds light on the U.S. Cadet Nurse Corps in Arizona. These stories ring true with one another. The insights developed through these encounters with other Cadet Nurses prompt me to tentatively conclude that similar patterns would emerge in the oral histories of other Arizona cadet nurses if their stories were known—but only to a point.

EDUCATIONAL OPPORTUNITY AND RACIAL AND ETHNIC DIVERSITY

It was remarkable (and arguably worthy of additional study) that a full decade before the civil rights movement started to gain traction, the federal government would be motivated to effect policy that required schools of nursing not discriminate by race, ethnicity or marital status in admissions practices. Previously, there were separate nursing schools for African Americans, and student nurses who married were routinely dismissed from nursing school. However, as will be discussed later, this idea to integrate nursing schools did not originate with the federal government; it was a response to political pressure exerted by those who were being treated unfairly.

There are a number of areas where it is not clear how successful schools of nursing were in enacting this policy instructionally or how successful the policy was being institutionalized into individual nurses' professional practice after they graduated. Admissions personnel in some schools of nursing were reluctant to change and comply; these schools were excluded from the Cadet Nurse Corps. The African American community exerted political and legal pressure to assure that this policy was part of the terms of the U.S. Cadet Nurse Corps and that these terms were met.[50]

Unclear is the degree to which the opportunity to graduate from high school—one of the requirements for admission to the corps—was evenly distributed in Arizona for those of Mexican origin who were not among the

300,000 to 500,000 forced out of the United States during the 1930s.[51] At the time, Arizona public education was segregated. It was not uncommon for Mexican-born and Mexican American children to be educated in one school and white children in another in the same district, and African Americans were segregated in Arizona, locating themselves predominately in areas like South Phoenix. Also at play was the well-documented discrimination in the workplace and military during World War II.

While a career pathway to the military was open to white women enrolled in the Cadet Nurse Corps, Maureen Honey, Cheryl Mullenbach, Darlene Hine and others reported that the door was not as wide open for African American women. Carey McWilliams and Robert Jones recommended improving the status of Mexican-born people in the Southwest who, because of more favorable experiences in the military than at home after the war, were beginning to awaken to and advocate for equity and fairness in the workplace and society. Similar statements can be made about the treatment of Native Americans as well. The existence of this uneven social and political playing field might raise the question among some of whether the nondiscrimination policy of the U.S. Cadet Nurse Corps could ever be fully realized on its own merit in Arizona or the rest of the country during World War II and the decades that followed. The messy, imperfect and decades-long efforts before World War II to professionalize nursing were the foundation on which Arizona's five participating schools in the U.S. Cadet Nurse Corps were grounded. Already underway in Arizona through previous generations of nurses and hospital administrators in Arizona were a process and structures to address the problem of discrimination and segregation. There was an emerging awareness that this gnawing problem was not going to go away on its own, and its continuation would not serve the country well over the long term. The nation's people were fractured, and they needed to be made whole.

In Arizona, the institutional mission of all five hospitals was to tend to the sick, regardless of religious affiliation or ability to pay. In at least two of the five schools of nursing, inclusion appeared to be already explicitly built into the mission of the school and hospital, or the school's mission targeted a particular poorly served population to the exclusion of others. Sage Memorial Hospital School of Nursing had a long-standing mission to the development of Native American nurses, and although the relationship between Clarence Salsbury and his counterparts in the federal government was frequently strained, nurses trained at Sage were sought out to work in BIA hospitals and clinics. Also, in its later years, the school opened to those who spoke Spanish and during the war to those who lived in the Japanese internment camps.[52]

Santa Monica's Hospital arose out of a community development project to improve healthcare for Latino, African American and low-income white people living in underserved South Phoenix. However, the federally funded public housing built in Phoenix under Emmett McLoughlin, which this hospital served, segregated Hispanic people, African Americans and low-income whites from each other. Also, Ruby Gordon reported that her class at Santa Monica's started with thirty-six students. Almost 20 percent of the enrollment was not white: three students were African American, one was Hispanic, one was Native American and two were Asian. In the newspaper article about Ruby's graduating class discussed earlier in this book, the Asian students were not even counted.

At the federal level, Estelle Massey Riddle, member of the Advisory Committee of the Division of Nurse Education and of the National Association for Colored Graduate Nurses, expressed concern about the low number of African Americans in the U.S. Cadet Nurse Corps. There were too few in relation to national needs and to serve the needs of the African American community, which at that time numbered some thirteen million. She was also concerned about educational standards for black nursing schools. "Although there is much improvement," she said, "there is still a policy to approve a school for Negroes on a much lower standard than for others."[53]

The Arizona evidence did not reveal how nurses of different races and ethnicities might have related with one another during or after the war. However, in the oral history of one of the nurses who was from the South, she mentioned how difficult it was to work with northern blacks. She knew blacks in the South and found the northern blacks disrespectful in comparison. In some subsequent work environments, she had no problems. What the story did not reveal was what happened that might have changed, either in this nurse or among the African American community.

Arizona cadet nurses working with Native American populations talked about cultural differences between them and Native Americans and how necessary it was to gain trust in order to work well with Native American patients. This is understandable, given the longstanding tension between Native Americans and the federal government, attributable in large part to the cultural insensitivity and lack of follow-through of the federal government.[54] Joan Douglas, a cadet nurse who trained at Stanford University and was a senior cadet among the Native Americans in Window Rock, Arizona, knew that she was forty miles west of Gallup, New Mexico, but made no mention of her proximity to Ganado, Arizona, where fellow Native American cadet nurses were being trained and whose graduates may have been working with or supervising her in Window Rock. There were an estimated forty Native American Cadet Nurses in the United States, which suggests that Sage Memorial, with thirty-two Cadet Nurse Corps graduates, may have been the primary producer of Native American nurses in the country.

It is hard to assert definitively that the U.S. Cadet Nurse Corps accomplished something that would not have been accomplished without this program because some seeds of educational equity appeared to already be taking root in the young state of Arizona but, again, only to a point. It is reasonable to assume that the infusion of funding and participation of young women in the U.S. Cadet Nurse Corps may have accelerated the initiation of a longer-term process of sea change in the nursing profession in Arizona, a process that continues to this day. However, details in the nurses' stories, when considered a generation after they were told, raise questions about the quality of the institutionalization of the U.S. Cadet Nurse Corps' nondiscrimination clause into nursing and nurse education during World War II and in the decades that followed. Having equal access to a high school education across racial and ethnic lines was not to be assumed during World War II. Also, simply being admitted to the program does not guarantee finishing the program of study. Not everyone who was a Cadet Nurse in these five schools of nursing became a nurse.

We should not view the past through today's lens, however. Such questions might be best addressed in consultation with cadet nurses trained in Arizona and not be limited to the stories of twenty-five, the majority of whom trained outside Arizona. This is an urgent concern because these women—now reaching their nineties—are rapidly disappearing.

The lessons learned during the 1950s told us that separate is not equal, but it is also important to remember that the curriculum of the 1940s was a response to previous decades and an author of the lessons of the '50s. The introduction of policies that require massive cultural change in any profession also take a long time to institutionalize into its culture. The U.S. Cadet Nurse Corps was a pivotal part of that curriculum, and the some 180,000 women who participated, of whom 124,000 became RNs, were essential actors in this normative process into the 1950s and later.

CROSSCURRENTS IN THE DESERT

The success of the U.S. Cadet Nurse Corps in Arizona was attributable in large part to the confluence of a number of key people both at the federal level and within Arizona. Many of the earliest leaders in the development of nurse education in Arizona in the early twentieth century—Deaconess Hospital's Lulu Clifton, Saint Mary's Hospital's Sister Mary Evangelista and Saint Joseph's Hospital's Mother Mary Paul—were women. In addition, during World War II, had it not been for Congresswoman Frances Payne Bolton, Surgeon General Thomas Parran, Director Lucile Petry and unanimous and swift congressional action, this federally funded program would not have gotten off the ground. Had such people as Dr. Clarence Salsbury, Father Emmett McLoughlin, Lulu Clifton and Sisters Mary Dominic, Mary Vincent and Mary Evangelista Weyand not been in Arizona to build what they established earlier, there might not have been an institutional presence with which to connect these federal resources. Finally, were it not for people such as Eleanor Roosevelt, who noticed gender, racial and ethnic inequities before, during and after the war,[55] the advances introduced by programs like the U.S. Cadet Nurse Corps might have been more difficult to sustain. It might also have been more difficult to sustain the momentum for change in the status of women in the workplace and at home that began to take hold in the '50s and '60s.

The U.S. Cadet Nurse Corps, similar to other federal programs introduced during World War II, prompted a continual flow of people, expertise and other resources into and out of Arizona, especially through the senior cadet phase of a cadet nurse's training. The effects of this effort were felt for decades after the war. At times, on the basis of this kaleidoscope of impressions, one can see streams of people of different races and ethnicities—military personnel, Nisei, Royal Air Force Cadets and cadet nurses, to name a few—moving from one place to the next within Arizona doing their daily business. Occasionally, their paths would cross, and the encounter would result in synergies that would yield outcomes greater than the sum of their parts. One such outcome reflected in the stories is the development of the School of Nursing at Arizona State University beginning in 1957. Another is the development and launching in 1965 of the associate degree program in nursing at Glendale Community College. A third is a collaboration at the Arizona Department of Health in cutting edge roles of the time of school nurse and school nurse practitioner. A fourth is the emergence of new approaches to healthcare among Native Americans. Yet another served her country in the military during subsequent conflicts in the 1950s and '60s and then served the military as a civilian nurse.

Such outcomes were revealed in about half of the twenty-five nurses' oral histories. The other half's stories took place on a smaller scale, in the context of the family and community. Cadet nurses whose careers were interrupted by family responsibilities told stories that showed the seeds of feminism. They ensured that their daughters were equipped for the changing world ahead of them, a world where the expectation that women stay home while men go to work would be less the norm. For this new world, women would need to be well educated. These nurses appeared to know this intuitively and only recognized the importance of this contribution in hindsight. (This message was one that I heard also from my cadet nurse mother, and for some reason, I heeded her advice.) These women were frequently the first in their families to achieve more than a high school education—at a time when young women were not encouraged to pursue higher education at all—and many were children of migrants as well.

The U.S. Cadet Nurse Corps, and its participants who were in or from Arizona, started processes in a metaphorical cultural borderland. These women were on the border between the norm of a hospital-based nurse education context revolving around the needs of the hospital and a university-based one centered on the educational needs of the student. They were also on the border between the norm of a woman's traditionally assigned role as wife, mother and caregiver and a modern self-determined role that also included pursuing educational opportunities and having a profession and career. Finally, the federal government, through the U.S. Public Health Service, was an actor in the awakening of many in the country to the need to begin the process to extend educational opportunity and health services equitably across racial and ethnic boundaries. None of these processes have been fully realized yet. This process is still very much a work in progress.

COMING OF AGE DURING WORLD WAR II

What do we know of the perspectives of other cadet nurses trained in Arizona, especially those of Mexican, African or Native American origin? What would their life stories reflect?

We normally associate World War II history with what is known as the "Greatest Generation," those born between 1900 and 1945 and who were the principle actors in political leadership and on the battlefields of Europe, North Africa and Japan. The elder siblings, born between around 1901 and 1924, were known as the GI Generation. Those born between 1925 and 1945 came to be known as the Silent Generation. Arizona cadet nurses were born during the mid- to late 1920s. They were the elders in the Silent Generation. Glen Elder and Kriste Lindenmeyer observed that the older GI Generation grew up in economically and socially secure times before the Depression, only to see their circumstances unravel when they entered adulthood during the Depression and World War II. The Silent Generation's circumstances were the opposite. They were born into economically and socially unstable times. As children they had nothing materially, and they came of age in a postwar era of abundance.

Cadet nurses in Arizona, as in the rest of the United States, grew up in an age when social ambiguities resulted in poorly defined identities for them as children, which stemmed from economic losses in nearly all social classes during the Great Depression and into the 1930s. Their families' economic losses led to an uncertainty of social status. This generation grew up in a progressive age; they were patriotic and trusting of the American government that had provided so much through New Deal programs. They came of age during a time when ambition and achievement were rewarded with power and status. The losses into which they were born caused the Silent Generation to overcome them through aspiration, setting goals and being driven by a purpose. In Arizona, however, unlike many other parts of the United States, the social context provided different sets of challenges to an even distribution of opportunity across the different cultural groups residing in Arizona during World War II. The war experience opened the eyes of Mexican Americans, Native Americans and Japanese Americans to long-standing social inequities that they had appeared to tolerate. Returning Native Americans and Mexican American soldiers, who had experienced equal treatment on the battlefield, found they could not continue to tolerate these historic inequities as they had existed in the U.S. Southwest. Over the decades since World War II, Japanese Americans also worked for reparations to compensate for hardship and material losses as a result of their involuntary incarceration simply because of a racist idea that their Japanese heritage constituted a threat to national security. This threat was found to be ungrounded.[56] The war also opened the eyes of Arizona's women. Cadet nurses, who unlike their sisters who worked in other industries during the war, emerged with a credential that empowered them to pursue a career in addition to assuming traditional female roles after the war ended.

The U.S. Cadet Nurse Corps program operated at the perfect time, one when so many young women were seeking new opportunities to satisfy the patriotic urge to serve their country through the noble profession of nursing. The U.S. Cadet Nurse Corps program emerged to serve an important and practical purpose in Arizona and the country. Many American men had died on the battlefield. This reality would likely affect how, who and when women would marry, if they married. For those who would lead part of their adult lives independently or whose income would be necessary to support a family, having credentials in a profession that would always be in demand would assure their financial security.

After World War II, Arizona's cadet nurses resumed the business of living their lives; many got married, started families and lived the American dream. Though with the Korean conflict came some anxiety about their future. For the most part, according to a 1951 *Time* magazine essay, young adults of this generation aimed for a good, secure job in a big company. There were no larger-than-life issues left to fight; getting on with a life that was not much different from those of their neighbors was the order of the day. Many young women of the Silent Generation started adulthood wanting both a career and marriage. Arizona's cadet nurses emerged from World War II with a credential that would support them in satisfying both of these desires.

In the same *Time* magazine essay, the following observations were made about the Silent Generation:

> *G.I. Joe's younger brother is better informed and educated, much better trained, and less sorry for himself. Maudlin cartoons today would not find the popularity they did in World War II. The AWOL rate is down, even the use of profanity has fallen off…"Little Joe" gripes about his officers, distrusts politics and government…He does not go in for heroics, or believe in them. He is short on ideals, lacks self-reliance, is for personal security at any price…*
>
> *The best thing that can be said for American youth, in or out of uniform, is that it has learned that it must try to make the best of a bad and difficult job, whether that job is life, war, or both. The generation which has been called the oldest young generation in the world has achieved a certain maturity…Young people most bitterly know the frightful cost of living to keep peace in the world, and they willingly submit to the cost, not from want of spirit, but from a knowledge that it is the best thing to do. You cannot say of them "Youth Will Be Served," because the phrase suggests a voracious striking out from security, wealth, and stability. The best you can say for this younger generation is, "Youth Will Serve."*

Mark Sumner noted that precious few statues and memorials mark the struggles of the Silent Generation and that we should not be silent in our praise and support of them. Coincidentally, the same has been said about Arizona's Cadet Nurses.

In her interview with Charlotte Katona, Joyce Finch brought up that the cadet nurses were an interesting group because more than any other group during World War II, they came out into the workforce when the war ended. She made the assumption that "about most of us…we were not going to do this forever, but for many of us it has been something close to forever." She continued, "Without cognitively planning it, we sort of look back and say, 'Gee, isn't it interesting how that worked out,' as opposed to young women entering their careers today who have a career orientation." Charlotte noted that there weren't as many career choices for young women during World War II, but the foundation that was laid for her through work experiences, tested and validated in a variety of settings, equipped her very well. She also pointed out that she was determined enough to succeed and that there were many people who thought it was too hard and that they couldn't succeed.

Charlotte viewed the U.S. Cadet Nurse Corps as a support to assist in the education of nurses for society. Consequently, she noted that she was very pro-funding for nursing education because, although it never covers all of the cost, it helps realize potential and provides incentive to continue. It is a support system that removes barriers to qualified people who need the support in order to succeed.

Joyce Finch noted: "I think, in the sense that there are studies that say, well this is what the government did and this is what it cost, but not what it produced, yes, except these numbers of graduates who finished programs between this time and this time, but not their contributions to society."

Did the U.S. Cadet Nurse Corps' nondiscrimination clause help promote equitable opportunity and access to high-quality nurse education in Arizona during World War II? It is hard to tell for certain, but it sure did not hurt. Did the U.S. Cadet Nurse Corps contribute to society? The evidence in Arizona points to a resounding, albeit qualified, yes.

EPILOGUE

At the beginning of this project, my intention was to describe what I thought would be limited to the history of a remarkable group of women in Arizona who participated in an important federally funded program. As I delved deeper into this history, I found myself taking a number of side trips into other aspects of Arizona history to find out more about the Arizona context. This background information would prove helpful in situating Arizona cadet nurses in a context where they might have had experiences with people who they would not have otherwise come to know during and after World War II.

As I reviewed historical accounts and archival information, the evidence appeared to indicate that during World War II, people in Arizona led their lives in socially or politically defined compartments. Japanese Americans were in two self-contained internment camps. Mexicans and Mexican Americans lived in close-knit communities in agricultural areas or near the copper mines or railroads. However, many Anglos in the U.S. Southwest appeared unable to distinguish between Mexicans and Mexican-origin people in the workplace. When they came into contact with Mexican Americans, Anglos frequently associated Mexican Americans—U.S. citizens—with Mexican braceros, who were viewed as unwelcome competition for scarce jobs. German or Italian prisoners of war also had their place, and cadets from Great Britain, China or Russia learning how to fly in Arizona skies lodged in yet another part of the state. Americans from across the country came to Arizona as well to learn how to fly in an inexperienced U.S. military force, and other people came to the state to provision the state's exploding defense industry. One can only imagine what it must have felt like for those pioneers who were already in Arizona when these waves of newcomers arrived. Some cadet nurses were among the pioneer families, and many arrived in Arizona much later. However, in reading and listening to cadet nurses' accounts, it appeared that their cadet nurse service provided for exposure to and mixing with people of different backgrounds.

Likewise, there was an array of interactions between these different groups of people. Mesa residents invited Royal Air Force cadets to their homes for dinner over weekends, yet about fifty miles southwest of Mesa were over thirteen thousand American citizens detained out of a fear that they might be unpatriotic simply because of their Japanese heritage. Native American peoples lived on reservation land across the state, and the federal government claimed some of that land for the internment camps, much to the chagrin of the Native Americans. Thousands of people going west to seek work during the 1930s and '40s flooded Arizona encountered large numbers of Mexican Americans; they also encountered Mexicans brought to the United States to address critical labor shortages in the West. The crops were at risk of rotting in the fields, and there were not enough hands to build the railroads or work in the copper mines. Just as people seemed to be unable to distinguish between the Japanese enemy and loyal Japanese Americans, so also the country seemed to be unable to distinguish between Mexican Americans and Mexicans. The terms of the U.S. Cadet Nurse Corps program prohibited Arizona's five participating schools of nursing from discriminating on the basis of race, ethnicity or marital status. Of the two of the participating schools of nursing in Arizona that met this requirement on paper, only one, Sage Memorial, had a long-standing history of admitting Native Americans and later Latinas and those of Asian origin.

Over the course of these diversions, I learned more about the history of five hospital schools of nursing than I had bargained for. Beyond the impressive work training Native American nurses in Ganado and launching an integrated hospital and school of nursing in Phoenix, there was a rich history of women in leadership roles in the development of the three other schools of nursing: Lulu Clifton at Deaconess Hospital in Phoenix, Sister Mary Evangelista at Saint Mary's in Tucson and Mother Mary Paul O'Grady at Saint Joseph's Hospital in Phoenix. These religious women were remarkable trailblazers at the close of the nineteenth century and during the first decades of the twentieth. None of these women came to Arizona with the intention of opening hospitals or starting schools of nursing. Clifton came to recover from tuberculosis, and when she regained her health, she decided to stay in Arizona to build a hospital because she saw a need. The Sisters of Saint Joseph and the Sisters of Mercy were teaching orders. They came to build schools, but Sisters Mary Paul and Mary Evangelista saw a need to be filled and directed their efforts to building and administering hospitals to serve the Phoenix and Tucson communities, respectively. The U.S. Cadet Nurse Corps was born into an environment where women's leadership was already established.

Through this research, I found a further reaching history about Arizona women and their persistence through adversity. Much of today's nursing practice in Arizona is the legacy of many generations of women and not limited simply to the efforts of cadet nurses. Some women were sent to the Arizona territory in the late nineteenth and early twentieth centuries out of a sense of divine guidance, and others came for more practical reasons. Many followed when the U.S. Cadet Nurse Corps program began. Through this book, I learned about many Arizona women who trained in Arizona, but Arizona's cadet nurses were but one current in a stream of generations of women with a variety of backgrounds and different ways of expressing their commitment to their profession and to Arizonans' health and well-being. Arizona's cadet nurses just happened to be in the right place at the right time not only in the history of Arizona and our country but also in the history of the nursing profession. They were pioneers in the nursing profession throughout their careers, and their legacy continues to be felt.

Arizona's cadet nurses lived and trained in a socially and politically complex and high-energy local environment. However, the accounts do not point clearly to evidence that shows that the cadet nurses were aware of this complexity or of the many actors in whose midst they were training and learning to be a nurse. Nonetheless, African American, Native American and Mexican American cadet nurses might have been more keenly aware of this diversity through exclusionary life experiences outside the Cadet Nurse Corps that white cadet nurses might not have experienced or noticed. This aspect of the U.S. Cadet Nurse Corps in Arizona is worthy of additional study, but as time marches on, firsthand accounts will be more difficult to gather as fewer and fewer cadet nurses are available. Regardless of their race, ethnicity or marital status, Arizona cadet nurses, as well as everyone else supporting the war effort in this state, participated out of patriotic fervor. I continue to be fascinated by this story and hope to capture more stories so that Arizona cadet nurses' legacy to the nursing profession and healthcare as we now know them is more fully understood.

Appendix A

THE ARIZONA CONTEXT

World War II P.O.W. Camps in Arizona

Base Camps	Population
Navajo Ordinance Depot, Coconino, County	250 Germans
Pima Prisoner of War Camp (Papago Park), Maricopa County	1,800 Germans
Branches	
Buckeye No. 1	530 Germans
Buckeye No. 2	530 Germans
Continental	150 Germans
Cotton Center	300 Germans
Duncan	200 Germans
Litchfield Park	850 Germans
Queens Creek	350 Germans
Roll (Yuma County)	unknown
Yuma (Yuma County)	350 Germans
Florence Camp, Pinal County	5,500 Germans
Branches	
Casa Grande No. 1	500 Germans
Casa Grande No. 2	450 Germans

Cortaro	300 Germans
Eleven Mile Corner	300 Germans
Eloy No. 1	300 Germans
Eloy No. 2	37 Germans
Maricopa	315 Germans
Mount Graham, (Graham County)	250 Germans
Safford (Graham County)	150 Germans
Davis-Monthan Army Air Base, Pima County	400 Germans
Imperial Dam, Yuma County	unknown number of Italians
Yuma Test Station, Yuma County	650 Italians
TOTAL POWs in Arizona	14,462

Source: Kathy Kirkpatrick, Prisoner of War Camps Across America, *2013.*

JAPANESE AMERICAN ASSEMBLY, RELOCATION AND DETENTION FACILITIES IN ARIZONA

	OPENED	CLOSED	PEAK POPULATION
WARTIME CIVIL CONTROL ADMINISTRATION ASSEMBLY CENTER			
Mayer Assembly Center, Mayer	May 7, 1942	June 2, 1942	245
WAR RELOCATION AUTHORITY CONCENTRATION CAMPS AND CITIZEN ISOLATION CENTERS			
Gila River Relocation Camp, Rivers	July 20, 1942	November 16, 1945	13,348
Poston Relocation Camp, Parker	June 2, 1942	November 28, 1945	17,814
Leupp Isolation Center, Leupp	April 27, 1943	December 2, 1943	unknown
U.S. ARMY INTERNMENT CAMP			
Camp Florence, Florence	June 1943	May 1946	343
FEDERAL PRISON			
Catalina Federal Honor Camp, Tucson	1939	1951	45 draft resisters

Sources: Jeffery Burton et al., Confinement and Ethnicity: An Overview of World War II Japanese American Relocation Sites, *1999, and Kathy Kirkpatrick,* Prisoner of War Camps Across America, *2013.*

Appendix B

IMAGES OF JAPANESE INTERNMENT CAMPS

Cadet nurses in Arizona resided and trained in a state that also included two Japanese relocation camps. These images illustrate the places from which a number of patriotic Americans came when they volunteered to serve in the Cadet Nurse Corps or in the military. These photos also illustrate the patriotic loyalty of Nisei demonstrated in these communities that arose not by choice but by circumstance. Some young women left these camps to become nurses, and neighboring hospitals outside the camps sometimes received residents of these camps as patients.

Appendix B

Photos of the Poston Relocation Camp

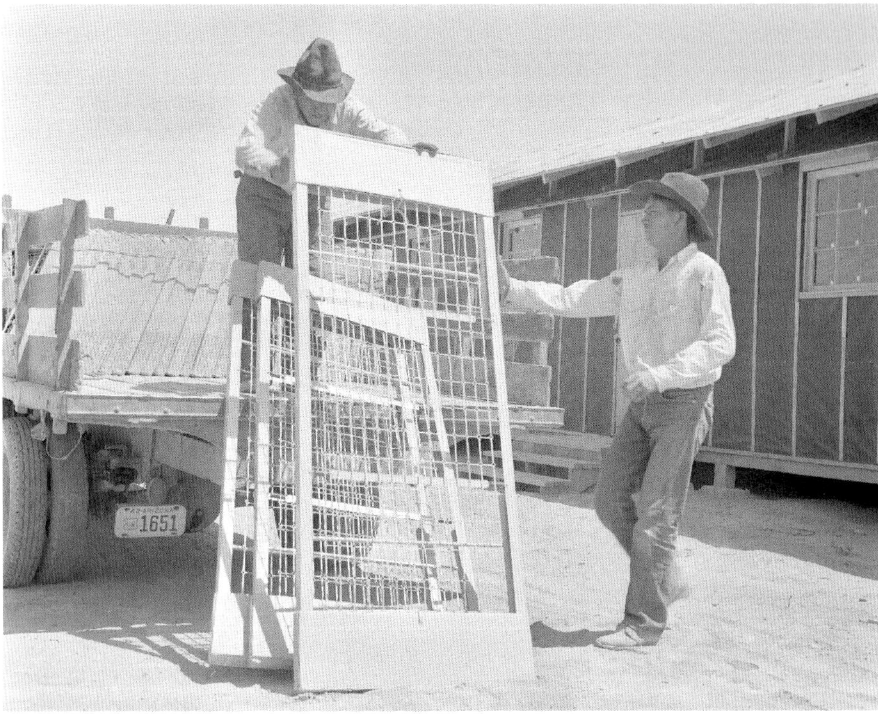

Apache Indians assist in the unloading of beds for evacuees of Japanese ancestry at this War Relocation Authority center, which was located on the Colorado River Indian Reservation. Poston, Arizona, April 29, 1942. *National Archives and Records Administration.*

Opposite, top: Construction continues on the War Relocation Authority center for evacuees of Japanese ancestry on the Colorado River Indian Reservation. Three units in the center are scheduled to house twenty thousand eventually. Poston, Arizona, 1942. *National Archives and Records Administration.*

Opposite, bottom: Aerial view of Colorado River Relocation center for persons of Japanese ancestry evacuated from the west coast. Poston, Arizona, May 25, 1942. *National Archives and Records Administration.*

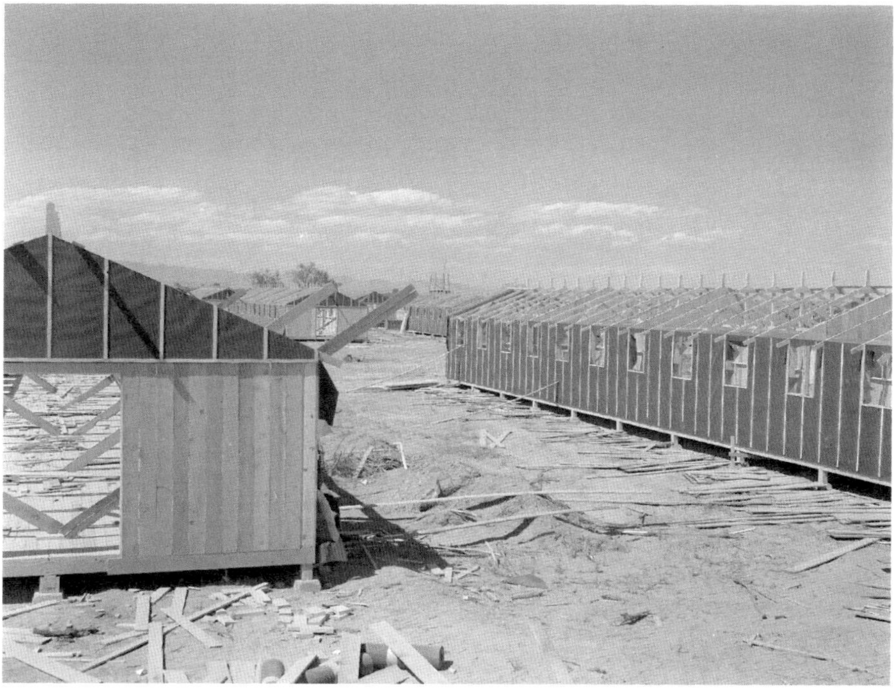

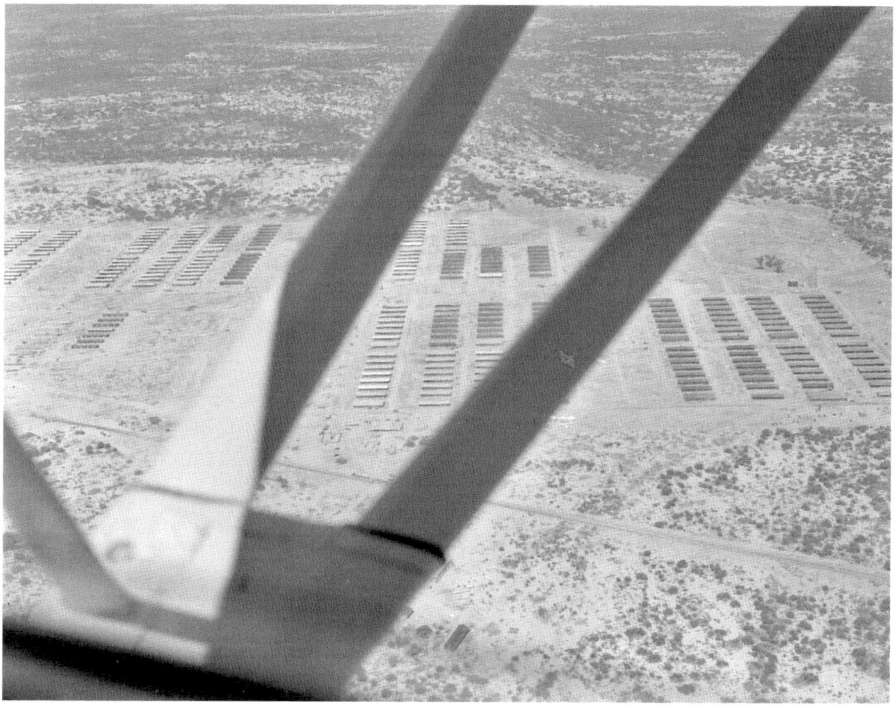

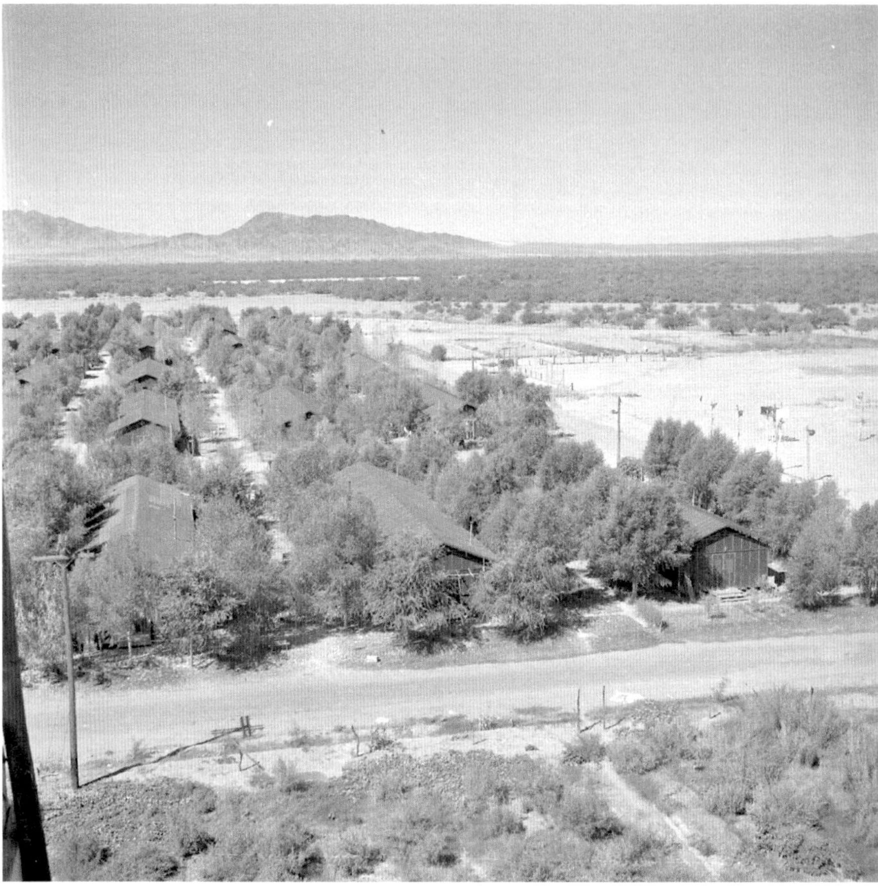

Although Poston, Arizona, was soon to be closed to Japanese Americans, it had already seen the beginnings of a new group of residents, the American Indians. On September 1, sixteen families, a total of seventy-eight people, came to Poston from the Hopi Reservation at Kings Canyon, Arizona. They moved into one of the blocks and seem to like it very much. Poston, Arizona, September 1945. *National Archives and Records Administration.*

Opposite, top: Mrs. A.D. Franchville, superintendent of Home Economics, on detail to Poston from Denver, Colorado, poses with a group of Hopi Indians near their new barrack-homes. Poston, Arizona, September 1945. *National Archives and Records Administration.*

Opposite, bottom: The Hirano family. *From left to right*: George, Hisa and Yasbei. Colorado River Relocation Center, Poston, Arizona, 1942–45. *National Archives and Records Administration.*

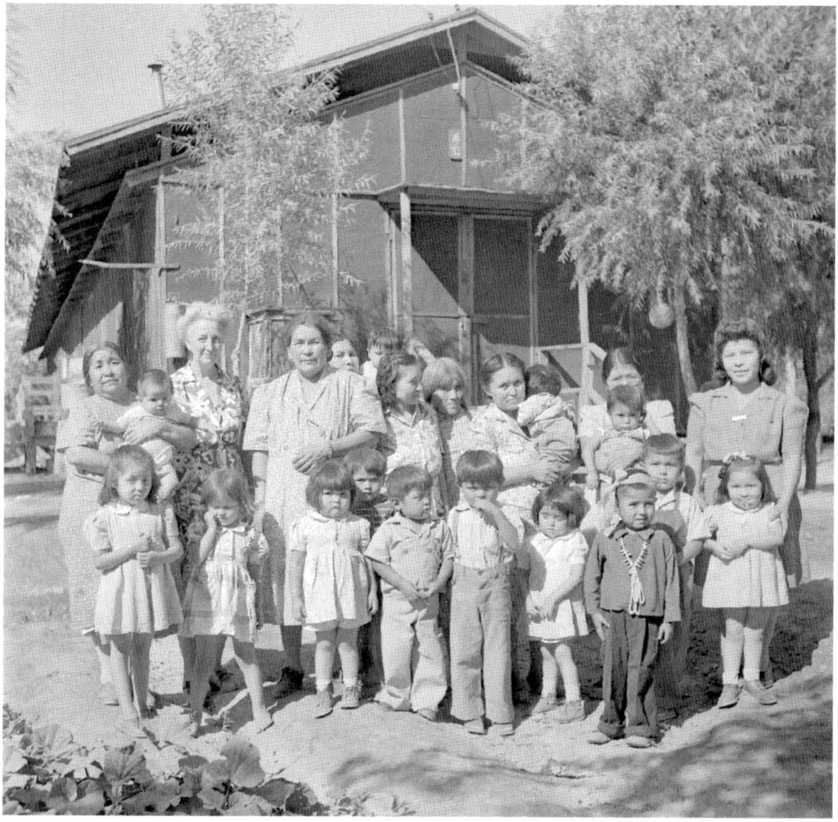

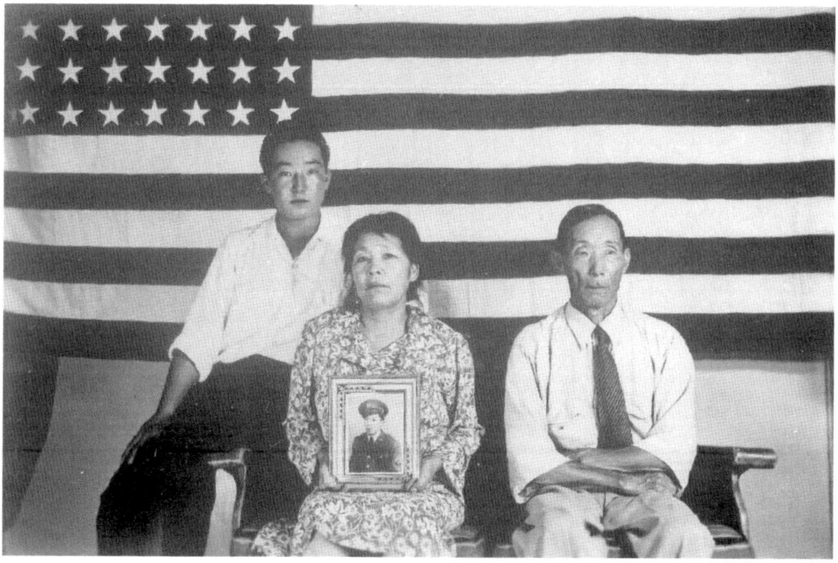

PHOTOS OF THE GILA RIVER RELOCATION CAMP

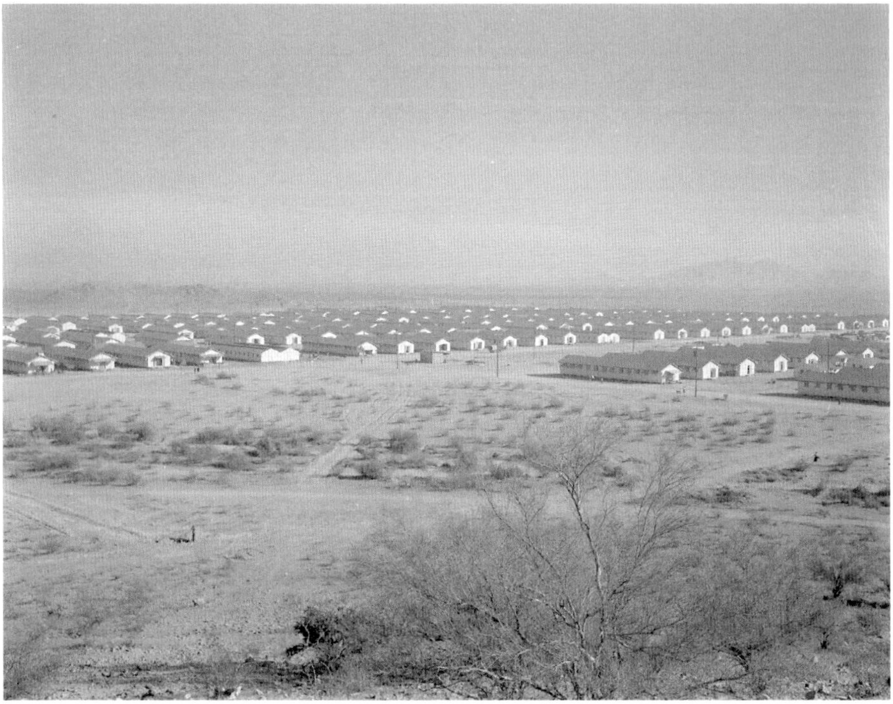

This shot shows a panorama of the northwest section of Camp No. 2. Gila River Relocation Center, Rivers, Arizona, November 27, 1942. *National Archives and Records Administration.*

Opposite, top: Butte Camp View. Gila River Relocation Center, Rivers, Arizona, March 14, 1944. *National Archives and Records Administration.*

Opposite, bottom: This image captures some of the school children who participated in the Harvest Festival Parade held at the Gila River Center on Thanksgiving Day, November 26, 1942. Gila River Relocation Center, Rivers, Arizona. *National Archives and Records Administration.*

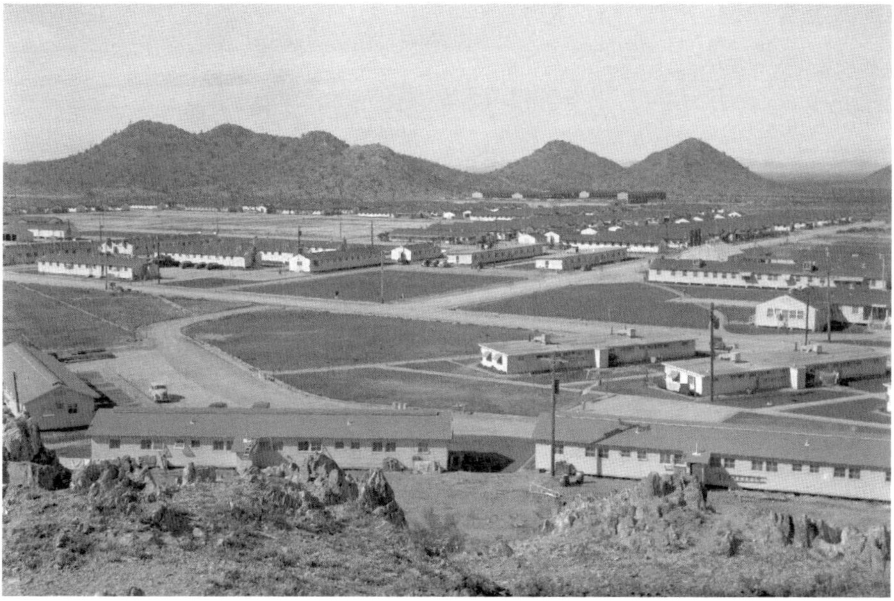

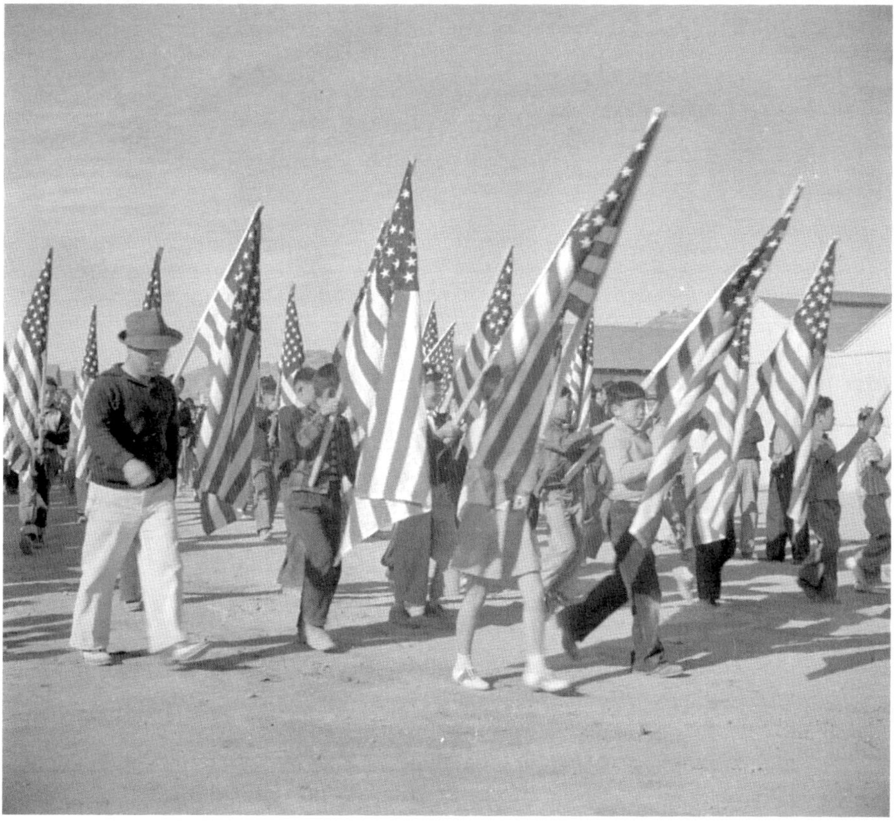

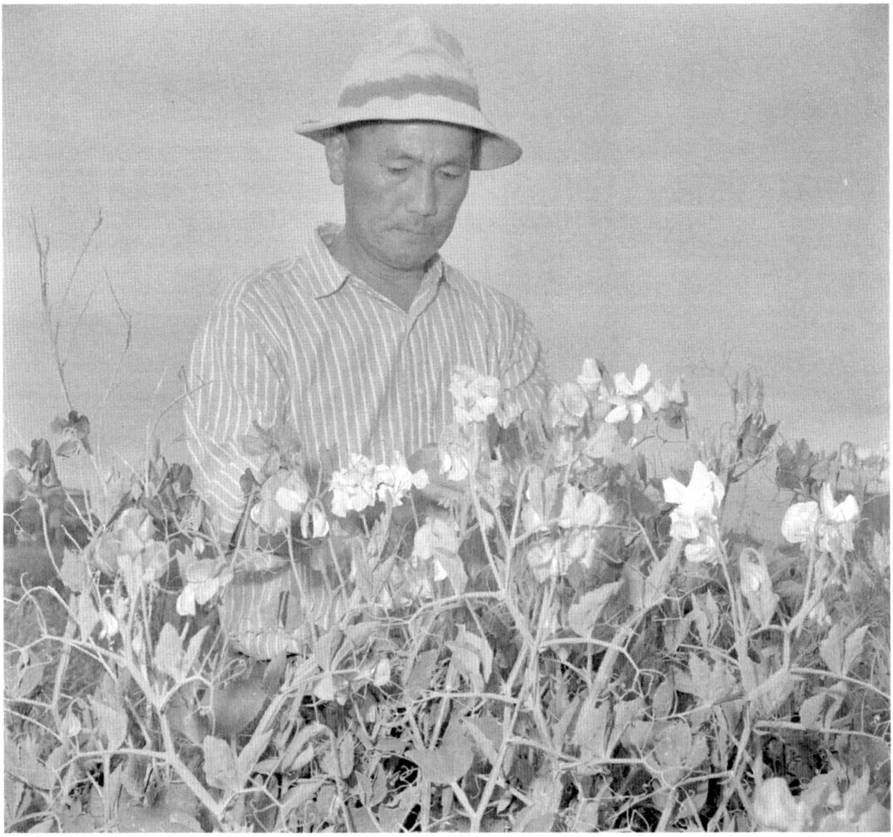

Paul S. Goya, former nurseryman at Sierra Madre, California, in charge of all flowers grown in the nursery here, is shown with a bed of prize summer sweet peas. He had been in the cut-flower business in Sierra Madre since 1921. Gila River Relocation Center, Rivers, Arizona, April 24, 1943. *National Archives and Records Administration.*

Opposite, top: Momoyo Yamamoto, formerly from Fresno, California, is shown here topping a large daikon, a large radish-like vegetable that is a great delicacy among the Japanese people. It is eaten either raw, cooked or pickled. The seed for this crop was loaned by Min Omata, unit foreman, from Fresno, California. This center harvested sixty-five acres of this vegetable and was the only War Relocation Authority project growing it in large quantities. Gila River Relocation Center, Rivers, Arizona, November 25, 1942. *National Archives and Records Administration.*

Opposite, bottom: Roy Katsura (left) and Haruo Yoshimoto check the superstructure of one of the model ships before the final assembly is completed. These model ships were used by the navy in a training program and were constructed by Japanese American craftsmen who wished to do their part in defeating the sons of the Rising Sun. Roy Katsura studied radio broadcasting operation in the National Trade School in Los Angeles, California, prior to evacuation. He had had no previous experience in model making, but his ability to use his hands made the training period brief. Haruo Yoshimoto, prior to evacuation, was a farmworker from Fowler, California, and had no previous experience in model making. Gila River Relocation Center, Rivers, Arizona, April 27, 1943. *National Archives and Records Administration.*

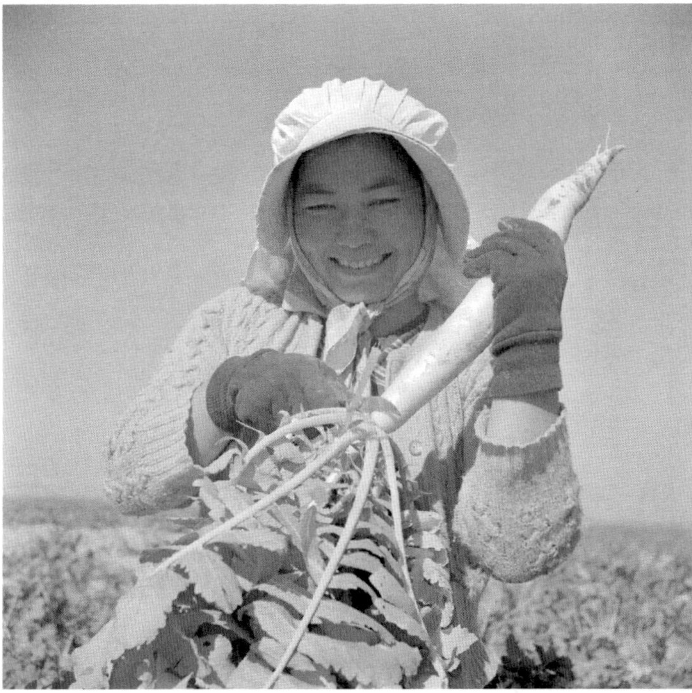

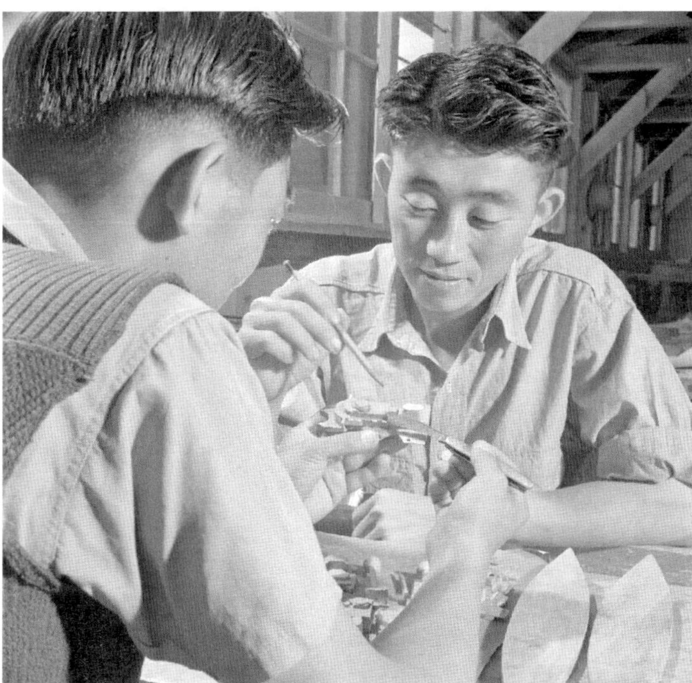

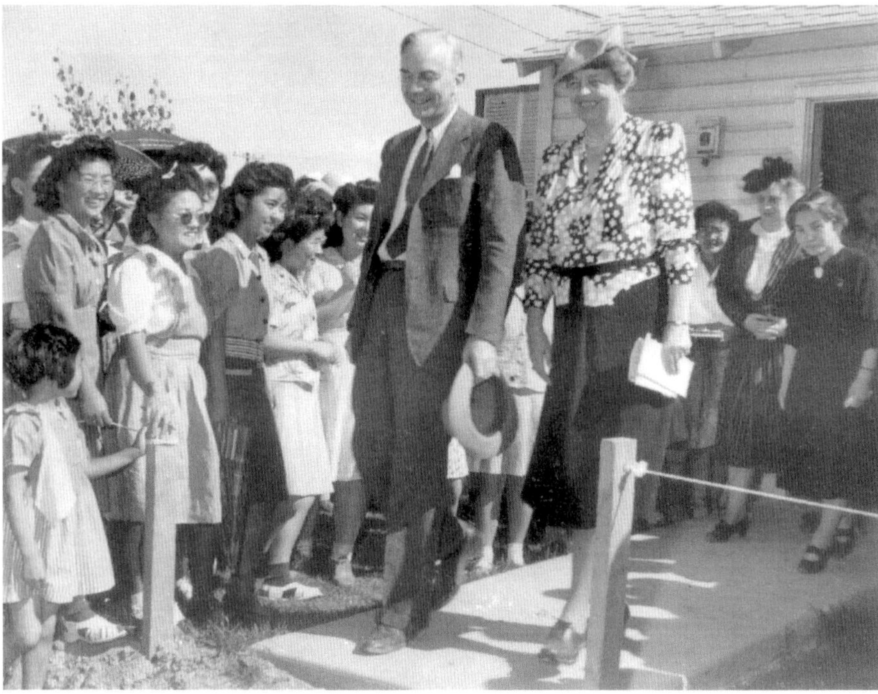

Eleanor Roosevelt at Gila River, Arizona, at a Japanese American Internment Center. April 23, 1943. *National Archives and Records Administration.*

Appendix C

U.S. CADET NURSE CORPS ENROLLMENT DATA

Students Admitted to U.S. Cadet Nurse Corps in Arizona, 1943–46

School and City	Number of Students Admitted	Percentage of Total
Good Samaritan, Phoenix	188	26
Sage Memorial, Ganado	39	5
Saint Joseph's, Phoenix	181	25
Saint Mary's, Tucson	226	31
Santa Monica's, Phoenix	98	13

Source: T. Robinson, Your Country Needs You. Cadet Nurses of World War II, *2009.*

Appendix C

Hispanic-Origin Presence Among 710 Cadet Nurses in Arizona Hospital Schools of Nursing

	Hispanic Surname		Percentage Hispanic Surname
	No	Yes	
Good Samaritan	169	7	4
Sage Memorial	24	8	33
Saint Joseph's	166	15	9
Saint Mary's	183	42	23
Santa Monica's	88	8	9
Total	630	80	13

Source: World War II Cadet Nursing Corps Card Files, 1942–48.

Appendix D

CADET NURSES TRAINED IN ARIZONA

Sage Memorial Hospital

Name	Date Admitted to the Corps
Winifred Analla	September 3, 1945
Virginia Ayon	September 3, 1945
Ana Marie Baez	July 1, 1943
Mary Louise Bayhulle	July 1, 1944
Elizabeth M. Brittian	September 3, 1945
Esther E. Candelaria	September 3, 1945
Lena Candelaria	July 1, 1943
Lillian B. Catcher	September 9, 1944
Ruthe B. Charlie	September 4, 1944
Elfrieda Conroy	September 3, 1943
Harrietta C. Curley	September 3, 1945
Sophie Davalos	September 3, 1945
Hazel Elk Head	September 4, 1944
Lillian V. Enos	September 6, 1944
Stella Garcia	September 4, 1944
Lydia Garibay	September 4, 1944
Naomi Garibay	July 1, 1944
Angela Garza	September 23, 1944
Rose L. James	September 3, 1945

Name	Date Admitted to the Corps
Lula Mae Kayona	September 14, 1943
Eleanor S. Letseoma	September 3, 1945
Grace Letseoma	September 5, 1944
Gloria V. Lewis	July 1, 1944
Leonora Lewis	July 1, 1944
Lillie Ann Maloney	September 1, 1944
Valentine Nuvamsa	July 1, 1944
Elizabeth Ortez	September 3, 1945
Evelyn Painter	September 6, 1945
Rowena Pentewa	September 1, 1944
Beulah Puckeshino	July 1, 1944
Neeley Rhodes	July 1, 1944
Frances Sanchez	September 3, 1945

Santa Monica's Hospital, Phoenix, Arizona

Name	Date Admitted to the Corps
Virginia Antone	October 1, 1944
Alta Marie Arpan	unknown
Ida Alice Bakke	July 1, 1945
Cora M. Baptisto	October 1, 1944
Verna Jean Becker	July 1, 1945
Eleanor Jean Bellanger	February 1, 1945
Elaine Ann Benson	July 1, 1945
Elisabeth Rose Marie Brown	July 1, 1945
Effie Dolores Brown	February 1, 1945
Isabel Bustamante	September 15, 1945
Dorothy M. Case	October 1, 1944
Betty Cavanaugh	October 1, 1944
Nellie Clarence	October 1, 1944
Mary V. Coats	July 1, 1945
Dorothy Gene Cooper	February 1, 1945
Ruby Juanita Daniels	July 1, 1945
Denice Jeanette Desjardins	July 1, 1945
Georgia Louise Dickson	September 15, 1945

NAME	DATE ADMITTED TO THE CORPS
Bette Yvonne Duncan	July 1, 1945
Margaret G. Ellis	October 1, 1944
Ida Lee Elkins	July 1, 1945
Cyrilla C. Endfield	October 1, 1944
Wanda E. Errigo	February 1, 1945
Jocie Kaneyo Eto	February 1, 1945
Dorothy Ferguson	October 1, 1944
Bonnie Dean Francis	February 1, 1945
Vera French	October 1, 1944
Vera Gilligan	July 1, 1945
Lois L. Glass	October 1, 1944
Virginia M. Godsell	October 1, 1944
Angelina Gutierrez	October 1, 1944
Patricia Ann Harrison	September 15, 1945
MaryLou M. Hext	October 1, 1944
Wyona L. Hinkle	October 1, 1944
Audrey Louise Hogan	September 15, 1945
Rose Marie Holden	February 1, 1945
Audree Io Holmgren	October 1, 1944
Gloria Beatrice Hudson	July 1, 1945
Dorothy Mary Jarvis	February 1, 1945
Clara Ann Johnson	October 1, 1944
Maria L. Jones	July 1, 1945
Mildred Jones	September 15, 1945
Mable M. Kayhill	October 1, 1944
Clarice Mae Lauer	February 1, 1945
Mary Elizabeth Lauer	October 1, 1944
Mary Jayne Layton	February 1, 1945
Ethel Louise Locke	September 15, 1945
Rosalie Theresa Locks	July 1, 1945
Lillian R. Maneth	October 1, 1944
Lucy B. Manuel	September 15, 1945
Ellazora Martin	July 1, 1945
Virginia Louise Mashaw	July 1, 1945
Julia Anne Mattill	July 1, 1945
Mary G. Milardovich	July 1, 1945
Gertrude Marcella Miller	September 15, 1944

Name	Date Admitted to the Corps
Lillian M. Miller	October 1, 1944
Verna Mockta	July 1, 1945
Helyn Lou Murphy	October 1, 1944
Clara Rebecca Nourse	July 1, 1945
Mary Ernestine Orr	July 1, 1945
Mary Joan Pappas	September 15, 1948
Virgie Lorene Parker	February 1, 1945
Carolyn Marie Peters	July 1, 1945
Floritta Genevieve Petite	September 15, 1945
Seymana Ethel F. Poleeson	July 1, 1945
Erma Anna Pollard	July 1, 1945
Rosalind L. Potter	September 15, 1945
Mabel M. Preston	February 1, 1945
Barbara Milton Proctor	February 1, 1945
Margaret Ernestine Ray	July 1, 1945
Lilly Reddy	July 1, 1945
Mary Ann Rodarte	October 1, 1944
Roberta Rosales	July 1, 1945
Flora Lee Rose	July 1, 1945
Jessie V. Ross	October 1, 1944
Blanche Sargent	October 1, 1944
Marian J. Sauls	October 1, 1944
Gwendolyn M. Schurz	October 1, 1944
T. Margaret Smith	October 1, 1944
Mildred Josephine Sneed	July 1, 1945
Stella Spencer	February 1, 1945
Mary Jane Stanberry	July 1, 1945
Evangeline Streeter	July 1, 1945
Mary Switenki	February 1, 1945
Uretta Thomas	October 1, 1944
Lydia Loreen Thomson	February 1, 1945
Margaret K. Thurman	October 1, 1944
Patsy Dean Trainor	July 1, 1945
Martha Jean Tuggle	February 1, 1945
Margaret Agnes Velasquez	July 1, 1945
Ruby Lee Etta Vinson	September 15, 1945
Barbara Wade	October 1, 1944

Name	Date Admitted to the Corps
Lois V. Wadlington	February 1, 1945
Regina Wender	September 15, 1945
Doris Edna Whinery	July 1, 1945
Evelyn White	October 1, 1944

Saint Joseph's Hospital, Phoenix, Arizona

Name	Date Admitted to the Corps
Lavon Aliver	February 1, 1944
Claire E. Altweis	unknown
Mercedes Alvarado	January 1, 1945
Dorothy Ames	February 1, 1944
Lucille Ruth Appleby	October 1, 1943
Jane Arnold	February 1, 1944
Jane Ashley	February 1, 1944
Jeanne Backs	September 3, 1945
Betty M. Bell	unknown
Margaret Benagas	June 12, 1944
Nancy Besch	February 5, 1946
Mary Ann Biegel	June 12, 1944
Martha Louise Bishop	October 1, 1943
Elizabeth Bishop	September 5, 1944
Mary Ann Bishop	September 5, 1944
Frances Borree	June 12, 1944
Betty G. Brazill	September 3, 1945
Wilma M. Broughman	February 1, 1945
Ruth Ellen Butterick	February 1, 1944
Katherine Byrne	September 3, 1945
Florence M. Cahill	February 5, 1945
Maxine J. Carpenter	February 5, 1945
Sara Mary Carr	October 1, 1943
Margaret E. Carr	September 5, 1944
Patricia A. Carroll	September 3, 1945
Tomasa Chavez	June 12, 1944
Catherine M. Chow	September 3, 1945

Name	Date Admitted to the Corps
Edna B. Christensen	January 1, 1944
Mary A. Claymore	September 5, 1944
Alice P. Cline	September 5, 1944
Mary M. Cole	September 3, 1945
Dorothy G. Cooper	September 5, 1944
Margaret Cooper	October 1, 1944
Barbara Courtright	March 1, 1945
Dorothy Cowan	October 1, 1943
Norma J. Cox	February 1, 1944
Shirley Fae Cremean	October 1, 1943
Joyce Crow	September 3, 1945
Virginia Davenport	September 5, 1944
Anna L. Day	September 5, 1944
Jacquelyn Lois Dewey	May 3, 1944
Mary K. Diederich	September 5, 1944
Norma Jane Ernest	October 1, 1943
Mary Patricia Fallon	September 3, 1945
Lillian Ferguson	September 3, 1945
Phyllis Finch	February 5, 1945
Rosita Flores	February 5, 1945
Margaret A. Flynn	January 1, 1944
Patricia K. Flynn	June 12, 1944
Sheila Flynn	February 1, 1944
Barbara Foote	October 1, 1943
Bonnie D. Francis	September 5, 1944
Florence Freestone	January 1, 1944
Ruth Freestone	January 1, 1944
Lucille B. Fricker	October 1, 1943
Pearl Golick	September 3, 1945
Lucia Rosa Gonzalez	September 3, 1945
Elaine S. Greco	June 12, 1944
Shirley E. Gustin	June 12, 1944
Alice R. Gutierrez	February 5, 1945
Catherine Hale	October 1, 1943
Mary Hall	June 12, 1944
Lillian J. Halvorsen	September 3, 1945
Bille M. Harman	September 5, 1944

Appendix D

Name	Date Admitted to the Corps
Oween Harper	January 1, 1944
Ernestine Hatch	October 1, 1943
Mabel Hendricks	October 1, 1943
Anne R. Hild	unknown
Aileen Holland	June 13, 1944
Louise Horne	October 1, 1943
Jean Marie Hudgin	September 3, 1945
Mary Carolin Hunsake	October 1, 1943
Ella Louise Hunt	September 3, 1945
Wilma Nell Jackson	February 1, 1944
Dorothy Mary Jarvis	June 12, 1944
Margaret P. Johnson	September 3, 1945
Thelda Ann Johnson	June 12, 1944
Margaret Anne Jones	February 1, 1944
Jeannette R. Kalisz	September 5, 1944
Joan Kear	October 1, 1943
Cynthia Anne Kendrick	September 3, 1945
Joyce Kimball	September 5, 1944
Janice Koesjan	June 12, 1944
Donna M. Kosin	September 5, 1944
Evelyn Lee	September 3, 1945
Foo Young Lee	September 3, 1945
Frances Jeanne Lewis	January 1, 1944
Eleanor Lively	April 1, 1944
Sue MacDonald	August 1, 1944
Margaret Emma Makin	September 3, 1945
Marion Louise Mara	October 1, 1943
Angelina Dora Martin	September 3, 1945
Eva L. Martinez	February 5, 1945
Herma Matyja	September 3, 1945
Nellie Frances McBride	September 3, 1945
Mary Jane McDonald	March 1, 1944
Edna McDougall	September 3, 1945
Sylvia R. McGettigan	September 5, 1944
Roberta L. McKellips	September 5, 1944
Dorothy McLeod	March 1, 1945
Helen Patricia Melby	February 1, 1944

Name	Date Admitted to the Corps
Donna L. Messimer	September 5, 1944
Helen Montgomery	September 3, 1945
Lucia Morales	February 1, 1944
Eva A. Moreno	February 5, 1945
Rosemary M. Mullen	September 5, 1944
Peggy Lou Myers	October 1, 1943
Josephine Navarro	February 1, 1944
Helen Newman	October 1, 1943
Bille R. Nunn	February 1, 1945
Kathleen M. O'Brien	November 1, 1944
Kathleen Louise O'Brien	September 3, 1945
Jane A. Olea	February 1, 1944
Madeline O'Leary	October 1, 1943
Mary K. O'Neill	June 12, 1944
Mildred O'Reilly	September 3, 1945
Marie Page	August 1, 1944
Dorothy A. Paxton	January 1, 1945
Patricia Perkins	September 5, 1944
Lorraine Emilie Pfaff	September 3, 1945
Ysaura Ramirez	February 5, 1945
Eleanor M. Regan	September 3, 1945
Ruth Richards	January 1, 1944
Betty L. Robbins	September 3, 1945
Ernestine E. Robles	May 5, 1944
Betty Jean Robson	October 1, 1943
Lupe Ruiz	February 1, 1944
Ilene Helen Ruybali	February 1, 1944
Jerry Eileen Ryan	February 1, 1944
Ellen Sanders	October 1, 1943
Mildred L. Sanders	January 1, 1945
Elizabeth Scherer	September 5, 1944
Nancy M. Schrantz	September 5, 1944
Jane A. Schuerman	November 1, 1944
Ruby Schuerman	October 1, 1943
Ann Sears	October 1, 1942
Mary Louise Seymour	October 1, 1943
Marjorie L. Sharrit	September 1, 1944

Name	Date Admitted to the Corps
Martha V. Sheehy	February 1, 1944
Mary Shestko	February 1, 1944
Madelyne D. Sipes	June 12, 1944
Leona J. Skaling	December 1, 1944
Rezella Smidt	September 3, 1945
Dorothy L. Smith	September 3, 1945
La Wanda P. Smith	February 1, 1944
Anne Srnanek	October 1, 1943
Barbara Stone	February 5, 1945
Joan M. Stout	September 5, 1944
Marjorie Taylor	September 3, 1945
Beverly J. Thomas	September 3, 1945
Lucille Thompson	October 1, 1943
Elma Thude	February 5, 1945
Sally Ann Thurber	October 1, 1943
Margaret E. Titcomb	October 1, 1943
Charlotte L. Tomerlin	September 5, 1944
Barbara A. Travis	September 3, 1945
Mary Travis	September 3, 1945
Helen Ruth Turner	October 1, 1943
Isabel Turner	September 5, 1944
Oral E. Turner	June 12, 1944
Dorothy Waggoner	October 1, 1943
Elfida Walker	September 3, 1945
Norma L. Walker	September 5, 1944
Roberta M. Warren	September 3, 1945
Frances M. Webster	September 5, 1944
Mildred K. Webster	September 11, 1944
Margaret Weddle	October 1, 1943
Mary Pat Weisel	January 1, 1944
Donna R. Whatley	February 1, 1944
Bette White	October 1, 1943
Cherrel White	January 1, 1944
Rachel Whitfill	January 1, 1944
Jacqueline Williams	September 3, 1945
Janette Williams	unknown
Lena Williams	February 5, 1945

Name	Date Admitted to the Corps
Patricia J Wilson	September 3, 1945
Nina F. Winninger	September 5, 1944
Mary Ybarra	March 1, 1945
Rosaline Zeilman	September 5, 1944
Ruth Zettel	August 8, 1944
Rita V. Zimmerman	August 29, 1944

Good Samaritan Hospital, Phoenix, Arizona

Name	Date Admitted to the Corps
Natalie Acuña	September 1, 1944
Marjorie Arnold	July 1, 1943
Norma Ashburn	July 1, 1943
Mary E. Ashby	February 15, 1944
Jane S. Avery	February 15, 1944
Mickey Babey	September 1, 1944
Margaret E. Bellah	February 15, 1944
Marjorie P. Benton	July 1, 1943
Angeline C. Bernklau	September 1, 1945
Angelina Bertaglio	February 15, 1945
Bonnie Bigelow	September 1, 1943
Dorothy A. Billasch	September 1, 1944
Aileen B. Blackwell	February 15, 1944
Betty L. Bloomstrand	September 1, 1943
Agnes Rebecca Bolden	September 1, 1944
Berta Roselynn Bruce	September 1, 1944
Mary E. Bryans	January 22, 1945
Wanda F. Burkhart	September 1, 1945
Betty J. Juncker Burwell	July 1, 1943
Barbara L. Busath	July 1, 1943
Frances J. Bushman	July 1, 1943
Mary Louise Campbell	July 1, 1943
Ora J. Campbell	February 15, 1945
Lucille B. Carlton	September 1, 1944
Rozan L. Carmichael	September 1, 1945
Mary L. Carney	July 1, 1943

Name	Date Admitted to the Corps
Elizabeth A. Carter	July 1, 1943
Rose Chavez	February 15, 1945
Deola Chesley	September 1, 1943
Jane Patterson Chowning	September 1, 1944
Mary Jane Colson	September 1, 1943
Geraldine F. Colvin	September 1, 1945
Georgia A. Combs	September 1, 1945
Sara L. Contreras	March 1, 1945
Elaine L. Cooper	February 15, 1945
Naomi L. Cosper	September 1, 1944
Betty Lou Craft	February 15, 1944
Patricia J. Craig	February 15, 1944
Margaret Ann Cronin	September 1, 1943
Carolee W. Crowder	February 15, 1944
Mary O. Davis	September 1, 1945
Rosie A. Ruvolo Denny	July 1, 1943
Dorothy A. Dull	July 1, 1943
Ada Eager	February 15, 1944
Lois Jane Ekman	July 1, 1943
Anita Esparza	September 1, 1945
Dolores A. Esquibel	September 1, 1944
Rosemary Farrow	September 1, 1944
Betty L. Ferry	September 1, 1943
Blanche Findlay	December 8, 1943
Jimmie J. Finney	September 1, 1944
Wanda L. Florence	September 1, 1945
Vera E. Ford	September 1, 1943
Amelia M. Fox	February 15, 1945
Dorothy E. Fox	July 1, 1943
Elise V. Freire	March 1, 1945
Jean M. Garrison	September 1, 1945
Rebecca J. Gay	September 1, 1944
Jeanette Gerhart	July 1, 1943
Francis B. Gibson	February 15, 1944
Della M. Glassgow	September 1, 1944
Gertrude Godbold	February 15, 1944
Dee Rene Gosling	February 15, 1945
Martha L. Hale	September 1, 1945

NAME	DATE ADMITTED TO THE CORPS
Barbara Hall	September 1, 1945
Elizabeth Hall	September 1, 1945
Elizabeth Hannum	February 15, 1944
Carolyn Harms	September 1, 1945
Prudy M. Hayne	September 1, 1945
Doris Heap	February 15, 1944
Esther J. Herrell	July 1, 1943
Jane Herrick	February 15, 1944
Margio R. Higgins	February 15, 1945
Dorothy M. Hilkins	July 1, 1943
Donna F. Hill	September 1, 1945
Elree J. Hodges	September 1, 1944
Claire Hoffman	February 15, 1945
Io A. Holmgren	February 15, 1944
Janet A. Hoyle	February 15, 1944
Betty R. Huebner	September 1, 1943
Katherine J. Hughes	July 1, 1943
Maude Ivanovich	February 15, 1944
Mary E. Jack	February 15, 1944
Phyllis V. Jensen	July 1, 1943
Ethelyn J. Johnson	September 1, 1943
Gaynelle Johnston	September 1, 1944
Marjory E. Jones	March 1, 1947
Ruth E. Jones	September 1, 1945
Elberta Kingsley Jonson	July 1, 1943
Thelma E. Journey	September 1, 1944
Catherine M. Joy	February 15, 1944
Rose E. Juncker	September 1, 1945
Marjorie D. Kennedy	September 1, 1943
Dixie Kiger	September 1, 1943
Dorothy L. Kilcrease	September 1, 1943
Maureen M. King	July 1, 1943
Edna M. Leeds	September 1, 1944
Elvera Lentini	July 1, 1943
Jean H. Lickerman	September 1, 1944
Doroty J. Lingren	September 1, 1943
Jeanne M. Long	July 1, 1943
Wilma A. Lounsbury	September 1, 1944

Appendix D

Name	Date Admitted to the Corps
Orpha C. Mauk	July 1, 1943
Nancy L. McAnally	September 1, 1943
Ruth McKee	February 15, 1944
Novice G. McReynolds	September 1, 1945
Rosemary Mealey	February 15, 1945
Joan E. Meek	February 15, 1944
Ruby M. Miller	September 1, 1943
Sylvia M. Mitchell	September 1, 1943
Beverly Morley	September 1, 1943
Harriet Mozinski	September 1, 1943
Katharine E. Nagel	July 1, 1943
Julie N. Rhoton Nelda	February 15, 1945
Thurza M. Orf	September 1, 1944
Virginia M. Patterson	February 15, 1944
Patricia B. Patton	February 15, 1945
Louise A. Perkins	September 1, 1943
Virginia Pierce	February 15, 1944
Norma J. Priest	September 1, 1945
Mary Irene Pyle	February 15, 1945
Mary E. Reed	February 15, 1944
Gladys I. Rencher	July 1, 1943
Phyllis F. Richardson	September 1, 1944
Glenna M. Riggs	September 1, 1945
Maria F. Rios	February 15, 1944
Elnora B. Roepke	September 1, 1944
Jennie B. Rose	September 1, 1945
Marion M. Schoenthaler	September 1, 1945
Opal L. Sexton	September 1, 1943
Maxine Shaw	September 1, 1943
Madge Shipley	September 1, 1943
Gertrude M. Shotwell	July 1, 1943
Edith A. Sims	September 1, 1943
Rachael O. Slayton	February 15, 1944
Dorothy L. Smith	September 1, 1944
Florence E. Smith	February 15, 1944
Roberta A. Smith	February 15, 1945
Virginia J. Smith	September 1, 1944
Lillian L. Solomon	July 1, 1943

Name	Date Admitted to the Corps
Leora C. Sorensen	September 1, 1943
Shirley A. Southworth	February 15, 1944
Veronica P. Stempin	September 1, 1945
Shirley A. Stratton	February 15, 1945
Frieda Suderman	July 1, 1943
Mary Suderman	July 1, 1943
Janice M. Swindell	September 1, 1945
Helen E. Taylor	February 15, 1944
Alene Thomas	September 1, 1943
Audrey L. Thomas	February 15, 1944
Joan M. Thompson	February 15, 1945
Helen Thresher	February 15, 1944
Sybil Thresher	February 15, 1944
Bette Ann Tirey	July 1, 1943
June L. Tryon	September 1, 1944
Virginia L. Umbaugh	February 15, 1945
Emma M. Vail	September 1, 1944
Nita M. Vaughn	February 15, 1945
Betty R. Voelker	September 1, 1943
Joan H. Von Rhein	February 15, 1945
Janet C. Vondracek	September 1, 1943
Lavera Waas	February 15, 1945
Eleanor J. Walmsley	February 15, 1945
Charlotte L. Warren	September 1, 1943
Ella M. Weiner	February 15, 1945
Mary L. Wilmoth	September 1, 1943
Christine Winchell	September 1, 1945
Mary N. Winkler	September 1, 1944
Jean H. Wittel	July 1, 1943
Ruth Wolfe	February 15, 1944
Zella W. Woodcock	February 15, 1945
Shirley Wright	September 1, 1944
Betty Ann Wylie	September 1, 1944
Eve Ziegler	February 15, 1945
Evelyn M. Zimmerman	February 15, 1945
Ruth E. Zimmerman	July 1, 1943

Appendix D

Saint Mary's Hospital, Tucson, Arizona

Name	Date Admitted to the Corps
Patricia M. Abbott	September 7, 1944
Loveda M. Ackley	January 21, 1945
Dolena Adams	September 1943
Mary M. Aginiga	June 18, 1945
Maria Aguilar	unknown
Marie M. Albanese	June 18, 1945
Geraldine Alexander	September 1943
Hazel P. Allen	June 18, 1945
Dora Anaya	September 4, 1944
Beatrice Anders	September 4, 1944
Stella S. Andrade	January 21, 1945
Jacqueline Jinnie Anich	September 9, 1945
Gloria Apodaca	September 1943
Louise Armstrong	unknown
Vivian Arnold	September 1943
Sara M. Autney	September 4, 1944
Mary Louise Avila	September 9, 1945
Barbara Joanne Barnes	June 18, 1945
Helen Ann Baur	September 9, 1945
Gwendolyn Beck	September 9, 1945
Mary L. Beck	September 4, 1944
Beatrice Bernal	September 1943
Alice C. Bess	June 18, 1944
Frances A. Bone	September 4, 1944
Jeanne Bowie	September 1943
Lois M. Boyce	June 18, 1944
Alice Elizabeth Briggman	September 4, 1944
Grace Brooker	January 1944
Rose Brozen	January 1944
Lenora Bryan	February 1944
Sara Eugenia Burke	September 9, 1945
Frances Burns	unknown
Irene B. Burrell	June 18, 1944
Beverly Jean Burt	September 4, 1944
Concha Cajero	January 1944
Lucille Cannon	January 1944

NAME	DATE ADMITTED TO THE CORPS
Lorraine Case	September 4, 1944
Bobette Cenotto	September 9, 1945
Joan Marie Childress	September 9, 1945
Betty Louise Circle	September 4, 1944
Betty Cirvice	September 1943
Marion S. Clark	July 1, 1944
Claribel Collie	October 1943
Darlene Addie Collis	September 9, 1945
Betty Jean Comstock	September 9, 1945
Ann Marie Courtney	June 18, 1945
Patricia Lucien Crane	June 18, 1945
Erminia de la Cruz	September 1943
H. Kathleen Curtis	January 2, 1944
Helen Czapar	October 1943
Dolores F. Delsid	January 21, 1945
Rose M. Dinovo	January 21, 1945
Betty Sue Doffern	June 18, 1944
Dorothy L. Dolan	September 5, 1943
Rita Dominguez	June 18, 1945
Ellen Donnelly	September 1943
Patricia Dougherty	June 18, 1944
Virginia Dowdle	September 4, 1944
Mildred Edgell	September 1943
Angelina Escobedo	September 4, 1944
Margaret Evans	June 18, 1945
Betty L. Farris	September 4, 1944
Dora Ethel Faubion	September 9, 1945
Margaret Firkins	June 18, 1944
Eleanor Fisher	September 1943
Mary Fitzgerald	September 1943
Dorothy Foley	September 1943
Gladys Jean Foley	June 18, 1945
Martha Franco	November 1, 1943
Natalie J. Friedman	September 4, 1944
Dorothy Fullerton	October 1, 1943
Rosalie Gallahen	September 1943
Vivian Guerrero Gallardo	June 18, 1945
Refugio Garcia	September 1943

Name	Date Admitted to the Corps
Naomi Gelina	January 1944
Marian Gibson	January 1944
Gloria Gil	September 9, 1945
Gloria Giron	January 1944
Ida Mary Giusti	June 18, 1944
Martha Glaser	September 1943
Margaret Glass	September 4, 1944
Roy Gobie	September 4, 1944
Marguerite J. Graham	September 4, 1944
Frances F. Guzman	January 21, 1945
Virginia Haffa	January 1944
Bonnie Harris	September 4, 1944
Geraldine Harris	June 18, 1944
Alida Margaret den Hartog	September 9, 1945
Patricia Haugh	January 21, 1945
Phyllis Heisterberg	June 18, 1944
Betty Hensel	January 1944
Madeline Lucille Herman	January 21, 1945
Ann Hillman	September 1943
Merle Hills	September 1943
Ruth Hoffman	September 1943
Helen F. Hogan	January 21, 1945
Norma L. Holaway	June 18, 1945
Mary Bernadette Hono	June 18, 1945
Molly L. Hooghkirk	September 4, 1944
Alice V. Huerta	January 21, 1945
Dorothy M Hughes	June 18, 1944
Margaret Hurley	September 1943
Sylvia Jiménez	January 1944
Ruth V. Johnston	September 4, 1944
Mary Jones	September 1943
Gladys Jane Junko	June 18, 1944
Carmen Jurado	September 1943
Carmen D. Jurado	November 25, 1944
Arlean P. Kagel	September 4, 1944
Marcella G. Korte	September 4, 1944
Miriam Krauch	September 1943
Doris Lane	September 25, 1944

Name	Date Admitted to the Corps
June Shirley Laning	September 4, 1944
Charlotte Lee Boff	January 2, 1944
Mary Elizabeth Leeka	August 1, 1945
Doris Loman	September 1943
Ruth Loman	September 1943
Cleo Maldonado	September 4, 1944
LaVerne S Marsh	September 5, 1943
Alice J. Martling	January 21, 1945
Mary Louise Mauler	June 18, 1944
Mildred R. McCool	September 4, 1944
Ardis McFate	October 1943
Barbara McGee	unknown
Margaret McGee	September 9, 1945
Mildred McMullen	September 1943
Gladys McNeil	September 1943
Elizabeth Jane Meers	June 18, 1944
Ruth Meloy	September 4, 1944
Hilda Merrill	September 1943
Eloise Marie Mescall	September 4, 1944
Agnes Miller	June 18, 1945
Eddene Miller	June 18, 1945
Lorraine Miller	September 1943
D. Louise Mitchell	June 18, 1945
Dalia Monreal	September 1943
Mary Evelyn Moore	September 4, 1944
Esther Morales	January 1944
Josephine Moreno	September 1943
Viola Mugford	January 2, 1944
Faye Murphy	September 1943
Lisa M. Myers	June 18, 1944
Margaret Nelson	September 4, 1944
Catherine Nichols	February 1944
Janet M. Nichols	September 4, 1944
Lola Norris	February 1944
Virginia O'Hagin	September 1943
Josephine Ortega	September 1943
Teresa Ortega	September 9, 1945
Rowena Elaine Otto	September 4, 1944

Name	Date Admitted to the Corps
Dora Packard	September 1943
Jean Paez	June 18, 1944
Jane Paquin	September 1943
Vera Paschal	January 21, 1945
Sabina J. Pesoti	June 18, 1944
Shery Philip	September 5, 1944
Viola Phillips	September 1943
Dorothy Piotrowski	June 18, 1944
Josephine Priscilla Pompe	September 9, 1945
Maxine Powell	September 1943
Mary V. Pringle	January 21, 1945
Sarah Marie Putney	September 4, 1944
Amalia Rada	September 1943
Marcella M. Ramade	September 4, 1944
Marcella Ramak	unknown
Bertha Ramirez	September 9, 1945
Carmen Ramirez	July 1, 1944
Josphine Ramirez	September 5, 1943
Adabelle Richardson	June 18, 1944
Barbara Ann Riddle	June 18, 1945
Lena Elizabeth Rigo	June 18, 1945
Patricia Robertson	June 18, 1944
Donna Robey	June 18, 1945
Mae Robson	June 18, 1944
Kay Helen Rodin	September 9, 1945
Lupe Rodriguez	February 1944
Anna Lee Rogers	September 1943
Mary Angela Rosselot	September 1943
Elizabeth R. Roy	June 18, 1945
Rosalee Russell	January 1944
Delia Salgado	September 5, 1943
Rosa R. Sanchez	June 18, 1945
Lenora Schafer	October 1943
Rosemary Schaub	January 21, 1945
Dorothy J. Schemks	September 4, 1944
Theresa Helen Schneider	September 9, 1945
Mildred Schulz	June 18, 1944
Phyllis Maureen Shaw	June 18, 1945

Name	Date Admitted to the Corps
Evelyn Slack	September 1943
Dorothy Slater	June 18, 1944
Isabel Smith	January 2, 1944
Audrey Stall	September 9, 1945
Eleanor R. Stewart	September 9, 1945
Bonnie Swindell	June 18, 1944
Mary K. Sykes	September 4, 1944
Lynette Tague	September 1943
Fae E. Teeter	January 24, 1945
Katherine Téllez	January 21, 1945
Noal Thomas	March 1, 1944
Dorothy Thrash	August 1, 1944
Clyda Lawrence Tisdale	June 18, 1945
Marjorie B. Tye	January 10, 1946
Lenore Vanover	September 1943
Frances Vear	September 4, 1944
Corinne Louise Vidano	September 9, 1945
Irene Walker	September 4, 1944
Henrietta Wallace	unknown
Melba Marie Watmer	unknown
Margaret Suzanne Wear	January 21, 1945
Maxine Weiss	unknown
Luella J. Welker	September 4, 1944
Frances P. Whelan	unknown
Mary Lee Whelan	unknown
Francine Wilhelm	unknown
Dorothy Evelyn Williams	unknown
Mary Ellen Williams	September 1943
Fleta Wren	February 1, 1944
Virginia M. Yates	September 4, 1944
Grace Zuick	June 18, 1944

Source: National Archives and Records Administration.

Appendix E

CADET NURSES LIVING IN ARIZONA IN THE 1980s

	Graduated	Arrived in Arizona	Estimated number of			Higher Education Level
			Children	Employers		
				Total	Arizona	
Career Practitioners						
Lucile Flores	1945	1946	2	12	11	Baccalaureate, 1949 (Science)
Charlotte Katona	1945	1981	2[2]	3	1	BSN, 1964
Donna Malone	1947	1979	3	2	1	
Leona Pearson	1944	1961	3	8	4	BSN, 1984
Jane Yettke	1947	1979	0[6]	13	2	
Hands-on Nurses						
Constance Besch	1946	1972	7	3	1	
Margaret Clements	1948	1972	2	9	4	
Katherine Day	1946	1952	1	9	6	Master's, ca. 1972 (Education)
Eugenia Dormady	1947	1972	9	6	1	
Betty Gerl	1947	1980	4	11	2	
Marylou Gertz	1947	1957	4	5	1	
Clara Gilmore	1947	1961	2	7	3	B.S., 1973 (Education with minor in health)
Bernice Green	1947	1955	2	5	3	
Shirley Kirking	1946	1975	2	7	2	
Doris Meharry	1945	1957	2	9	3	

June Niccum	1948	1973	4	7	1	BSN, 1981
Elaine Sabel	1947	1973	2[2]	6	3	
Nurse and Public Health Education leaders						
Ellie Branstetter	1944[1,5]	1945	0	7	6	Ph.D. 19693
Joan Douglas	1945	1980	0	7	1	Master's, 1959 (Public Health)
Ruby Gordon	1948	Before 1948	1	9	9	Ph.D., 1975 (Adult Education and Administration)
Rosemary Johnson	1946	1959	0[1]	7	1	MSN, 1958 (Public Health Nursing and Community Mental Health) Ph.D., ABD4
Elaine Katzman	1948	1982	3	10	1	Ph.D., ca. 1984 (Family Studies)
Frances Knudsen	1946	1951	5	4	3	Ph.D., 1979 Master's, 1964
Georgia Macdonough	1947	1963	3	9	3	Master's, 1968 (Counseling Education)
Barbara Miller	1947	1975	2	5	1	Ph.D., 1984 (Educational Administration)
TOTALS:			65	180	74	

Source: Joyce Finch Oral History Project

Notes: 1) Neither Rosemary Johnson nor Ellie Branstetter married; 2) Estimated minimum number of children; 3) No specialization mentioned; Ellie Branstetter's master's degree was in public health and nursing; 4) Rosemary Johnson studied at UCLA but was unable to complete the dissertation because of the death of her chair and other professional reasons; 5) Ellie Branstetter started nursing school before the U.S. Cadet Nurse Corps was established; 6) Jane Yettke's husband had a child from a previous marriage.

NOTES

1. See Goldmark, *Nursing and Nursing Education in the United States*, 1923.
2. U.S. Public Law 74.
3. U.S. House of Representatives, *Recruitment and Training of Nurses*.
4. WNET, "Frances Payne Bolton."
5. U.S. Public Law 76-849.
6. Kalisch and Kalisch. "Be a Cadet Nurse," 444–49.
7. See Product Advertising section in *How Advertisers Can Cooperate with the U.S. Cadet Nurse Corps*, 1943
8. Ibid.
9. Inserted in the 1942 packet were Cecilia L. Schulz's "White Caps—First Aides to Our Fighting Forces," reprinted from the Career Department section of the 1942 issue of *Mademoiselle Magazine*, which would appeal to high school students. Dorothy Dunbar Bromley's "A Career for College Girls," reprinted from the June 1942 *Harper's Magazine*, would engage young college women. In "The Nursing Profession and the War Effort," Katharine Faville proposed that if men were expected to leave well-paying positions to go to war, then women needed to step up and become the nurses who would be needed to care for them. She also indicated that the argument went further: when the war was over, the nurse's skills would be in just as great, if not greater, demand. In 1942, the year before the beginning of the U.S. Cadet Nurse Corps, money was frequently cited as an obstacle to becoming a student nurse.
10. See National Committee for War Service "Recruitment of Student Nurses," 2.

11. Furman and Williams, *Profile of the United States Public Health Service.*
12. U.S. Public Health Service, *United States Cadet Nurse Corps.*
13. Kalisch and Kalisch, *Federal Influence and Impact on Nursing.*
14. Carlos Vélez-Ibáñez has written extensively on this topic in a number of publications, notably *Border Visions*, University of Arizona Press, 1996. In her 1993 article titled "Mexican Americans on the Home Front: Community Organization in Arizona during World War II," Christine Marin wrote about the emergence of Mexican and Mexican American community organizations in Arizona during World War II. The appearance of these organizations was due in part to exclusionary practices enacted by existing organizations among the broader community.
15. See McWilliams to Rockefeller, 12. McWilliams described a Mexico that lay within the United States, made up of a Mexican population in Texas, New Mexico, Colorado, Arizona and California. Some are U.S. citizens, and others are not. He characterized this population as torn by conflicting loyalties and allegiances to both the United States and Mexico. McWilliams proposed that the U.S. national government "demonstrate its good will by taking immediately feasible steps to improve the social, economic, and political status of this group and, of course, to publicize this fact widely throughout Latin America."

    Robert Jones's *Mexican War Workers in the United States* was commissioned by the Division of Labor and Social Information, Pan American Union, in 1945. In his evaluation of what is commonly known as the Bracero program, Jones described a similar tense relationship between Mexican migrant workers in the U.S. Southwest and their employers in agriculture and the railroad industry, where, during both world wars, there was a critical labor shortage. Contract terms were not always followed by employers. Mexican migrants came to the United States for a number of reasons, including a deep sense of patriotism, as well as to learn new skills to bring back with them to Mexico, to improve their own economic status and to become conversant in English. Instead, they found themselves not receiving these federally funded and agreed-upon benefits during their stay in the United States.
16. Stanford University history professor Daniel Kennedy made this observation in the TV documentary *World War II from Space*, which was aired by the History Channel in 2012.
17. See Kirkpatrick, *Prisoner of War Camps Across America.*
18. See Robinson, *Nisei Cadet Nurse of World War II.*
19. Ibid.

20. Ibid., *Your Country Needs You.*
21. See Melton and Smith, *Arizona Goes to War.*
22. Davies, *Healing Ways.*
23. Trennert, "Sage Memorial Hospital," 353–74.
24. Ibid., *White Man's Medicine*; Davies, *Healing Ways.*
25. Kristofic, "Building Bridges Between Old and New."
26. Pollitz, Streeter and Walsh, "Nurse's Journey."
27. Robinson, *Your Country Needs You.*
28. Pascoe, *Relations of Rescue*; ibid., "Western Women at the Cultural Crossroads," 40–58.
29. Shields, *White Caps in the Desert.*
30. Ibid., 63.
31. See Todd-Allard, "Miracle on 7th Avenue," for more information about Father Emmett's efforts in developing the South Phoenix community and addressing the healthcare shortage there.
32. Ibid.
33. Roosevelt, "My Day"; also cited in Luckingham, *Minorities in Phoenix*, 155.
34. Thelma Robinson estimated 98 graduates in *Your Country Needs You*, and Shields reported 145 graduates in *White Caps in the Desert.*
35. National League for Nursing Education, *Standard Curriculum.*
36. Ames, *History of the School of Nursing*; Randolph, "History of Regulation," 6, 8; Ridenour, "Arizona State Board of Nursing," 4.
37. As reported in Ames, *History of the School of Nursing*, 14.
38. Ancestry.com, World War II Cadet Nursing Corps Card Files.
39. U.S. Public Health Service, *United States Cadet Nurse Corps.*
40. Joyce Finch Collection. Professor Finch also reported on these oral histories at the annual conference of the American Association for the History of Nursing in 1988.
41. U.S. Public Health Service, *United States Cadet Nurse Corps*; Robinson, *Your Country Needs You.*
42. The Comprehensive Employment and Training Act was a U.S. federal law signed by President Richard Nixon on December 28, 1973, to train workers and provide them with jobs in public service. The program offered work to the long-term unemployed and those with low incomes. Full-time jobs were provided for a period of twelve to twenty-four months in public agencies or private nonprofit organizations. The intent was to impart a marketable skill that would allow participants to move to an unsubsidized job. It was an extension of the Works Progress Administration program from the 1930s.

43. I learned of Sylvia Jiménez Almeyda through personal communication with Christine Marin on February 5, 2014, and through her U.S. Cadet Nurse Corps membership card. This description is an almost verbatim transcript of Christine's recollection of her neighbor and good friend.
44. Kuehneman, "Sylvia Jiménez Almeyda."
45. Ibid.
46. Ibid.
47. Cadet Nurses' Legacy to Nursing.
48. For example: Pursglove, oral history interview by Hannah Fisher; Robinson, *Nisei Cadet Nurse of World War II*; and Robinson and Perry, *Cadet Nurse Stories*. There are a growing number of cadet nurse oral histories archived in a number of online repositories, including eighty-three cadet nurse oral histories in the Library of Congress Veterans History Project (http://lcweb2.loc.gov/diglib/vhp/search?query=cadet+nurse+corps&field=all), four cadet nurse oral histories among the many resources at the University of North Carolina–Greensboro's Betty H. Carter Women Veterans Historical Project (http://libcdm1.uncg.edu/cdm/search/collection/WVHP/searchterm/cadet%20nurse%20corps/field/servic/mode/all/conn/and/order/date/page/2) and one cadet nurse oral history at the Voces Oral History Project at the University of Texas–Austin (http://www.lib.utexas.edu/voces/template-stories-indiv.html?work_urn=urn%3Autlol%3Awwlatin.539&work_title=Gonzalez%2C+Florence). Oral histories of cadet nurses can also be found in other archives, such as the Oregon Health and Science University; the Boulder, Colorado Public Library; and the Minnesota State University–Mankato South Central Minnesota Veterans History Project. Archives like these are good locations to house additional cadet nurse oral histories; I have become acquainted with a number of cadet nurses' children, now themselves of retirement age, through the uscadetnurse.org website and through luncheons honoring cadet nurses' legacies in Bethesda, Maryland, and Quincy, Massachusetts.
49. *Mendocino Beacon*, obituary of Ana Marie Bruenger; *Payson Roundup*, obituary of Clara Rebecca Nourse Sumpter.
50. See U.S. Public Health Service, *United States Cadet Nurse Corps*, and Clark Hine, *Black Women in White*, for discussion of African American women's participation in the U.S. Cadet Nurse Corps. See also Henderson, "Better and Greater Service for Humanity," and Staupers, *No Time for Prejudice*, for discussion of the National Association of Colored Graduate Nurses' (NACGN) role in the professionalization of black nursing and pressing

for integration in civilian and military nursing. The NACGN dissolved in 1949, and its members folded into the American Nursing Association when it was apparent that its purpose had been served.

51. See the video "Deportation" on WETA and Latino Public Television, *Latino Americans*, http://www.pbs.org/latino-americans/en/watch-videos/#2365053363.

52. Salsbury with Hughes, *Salsbury Story*; Trennert, "Sage Memorial Hospital," 353–74.

53. U.S. Public Health Service, *United States Cadet Nurse Corps*, 50.

54. Trennert, "Sage Memorial Hospital," 353–74; ibid., *White Man's Medicine*; Davies, *Healing Ways*; Salsbury with Hughes, *Salsbury Story*.

55. As early as 1939, when she resigned from the Daughters of the American Revolution for their refusal to permit Marian Anderson to sing at Constitution Hall in Washington, D.C., Eleanor Roosevelt was aware of and a champion for change to end racial and ethnic discrimination in the United States. After World War II, she was the U.S. ambassador to the United Nations and was instrumental in the drafting of the U.N. Declaration of Human Rights.

56. See National Park Service, "Personal Justice Denied."

BIBLIOGRAPHY

Archival Sources

Ancestry.com. World War II Cadet Nursing Corps Card Files, 1942–48. Provo, UT: Ancestry.com Operations, Inc. Original data: Cadet Nurse Corps Files, compiled 1943–48, documenting the period 1942–48. MLR Number: UD-WW 10; ARC ID: 5605027; 350 boxes. Records of the Public Health Service, 1794–1990, Record Group 90. Washington, D.C.: National Archives, 2011.

Gonzales González, Telesfora Barbara. Oral history interview by Raquel C. Garza and Emily Cox, August 2, 2006. San Antonio, Texas. Voces Oral History Project. University of Texas–Austin. http://www.lib.utexas.edu/voces/template-stories-indiv.html?work_urn=urn%3Autlol%3Awwlatin.539&work_title=Gonzalez%2C+Florence.

Guzman, Henry M. "Transition and Emergence: Mexican-Americans in the Border States, 1930–1950." Unpublished paper, 1992.

History of Good Samaritan Hospital School of Nursing. Binder 1. Drawer 4. Banner Good Samaritan Hospital Archival Collection.

Joyce Finch Collection. Tempe, AZ: College of Nursing, Arizona State University, 1987.

McWilliams, Carey, to Nelson Rockefeller, October 15, 1941. Box 27. Carey McWilliams Papers (1243). Young Research Library, Los Angeles, California.

Pursglove, Blanche. Oral history interview by Hannah Fisher, June 24, 1989. Tape recording. Brownsville, Pennsylvania.

PUBLISHED SOURCES

Ames, Mary Aloysia. *History of the School of Nursing, 1914–1966: St. Mary's Hospital, Tucson*. Tucson: Arizona Pioneers' Historical Society, 1966.

Arizona Republic. "Here's How 112,000 Cadet Nurses Are Serving in Hospitals Now: Take This Opportunity to Enlist in This Proud Profession." N.d.

———. "Santa Monica's Hospital Will Graduate 21: Second Inter-Racial Class Exercises Due Thursday." June 27, 1948.

Arizona Republican. "St. Joseph's Hospital One of the Most Complete in Southwest." December 31, 1922, 4. ProQuest Historical Newspapers.

Burton, Jeffrey F., Mary M. Farrell, Florence B. Lord and Richard W. Lord. *Confinement and Ethnicity: An Overview of World War II Japanese American Relocation Sites*. Tucson, AZ: Western Archeological and Conservation Center, National Park Service, U.S. Department of the Interior, 1999.

Cadet Nurses' Legacy to Nursing. uscadetnurse.org. 2011–16.

Clark Hine, Darlene. *Black Women in White: Racial Conflict and Cooperation in the Nursing Profession, 1890–1950*. Bloomington: University of Indiana Press, 1989.

Committee on Recruitment of Student Nurses. "Recruitment of Student Nurses: Material for State and Local Committees." New York: National Nursing Council for War Service, 1942.

Davies, Wade. *Healing Ways: Navajo Health Care in the Twentieth Century*. Albuquerque: University of New Mexico Press, 2001.

Dawson, Jim. *The RAF in Arizona Falcon Field, 1941–1945*. Newnan, GA: Stenger-Scott Publishing, 2002.

Densho Encyclopedia. http://encyclopedia.densho.org. 2012.

Elder, Glen. *Children of the Great Depression: Social Change in Life Experience*. Chicago: University of Chicago Press, 1974.

Finch, Joyce. "Contributions of Cadet Nurses: An Oral History: 1943–1987." Abstract of paper presented at the Fifth-Annual Fall Conference on Nursing History of the American Association for the History of Nursing and College of Nursing and Health, University of Cincinnati, September 1988.

Franklin, Kathy Smith. "'A Spirit of Mercy': The Founding of Saint Joseph's Hospital, 1892–1912." Master's thesis, Arizona State University, 1997.

Furman, Bess, and Ralph Williams. *A Profile of the United States Public Health Service, 1798–1948*. Bethesda, MD: U.S. Department of Health, Education and Welfare, National Institutes of Health, 1973.

Goldmark, Josephine Clara, chair. Committee for the Study of Nursing Education. *Nursing and Nursing Education in the United States*. New York: J.J. Little & Ives Company. 1923.

Henderson, Lindsey. "Better and Greater Service for Humanity: The National Association of Colored Graduate Nurses and Integration in Nursing." Senior thesis, University of North Carolina–Asheville, 2013.

Honey, Maureen, ed. *Bitter Fruit: African American Women in World War II*. Columbia: University of Missouri Press, 1999.

Jones, Robert C. *Mexican War Workers in the United States*. Washington, D.C.: Pan American Union, 1945.

Kalisch, Philip A., and Beatrice J. Kalisch. *The Advance of American Nursing*. 3rd ed. Philadelphia: Lippincott, 1995.

———. "Be a Cadet Nurse: The Girl with a Future." *Nursing Outlook* 21, no. 7 (1973): 444–49.

———. *The Federal Influence and Impact on Nursing*. Hyattsville, MD: U.S. Department of Health and Human Services, Public Health Service, Health Resources Administration, Bureau of Health Professions, Division of Nursing, 1980.

Kingman Mohave Miner. "Tucson High School Girls to Enter Cadet Nurse Corps." April 25, 1945.

Kirkpatrick, Kathy. *Prisoner of War Camps Across America*. Salt Lake City, UT: Gentracer, 2013.

———. "Prisoners of World War II in the USA." Gentracer, 2015.

Kristofic, Jim. "Building Bridges Between Old and New." *Navajo Times*, 2009. http://navajotimes.com/entertainment/2009/1109/112509bridges.php.

———. "'Flying Lady' Adele Slivers." *Native Peoples Magazine* 25, no. 3 (2012): 52.

Kuehneman, Ed. "Sylvia Jiménez Almeyda, Cadet Nurse Corps." *Copper Canyon News*, August 3, 2010. http://www.coppercountrynews.com/v2_news_articles.php?heading=0&story_id=1371&pa.

Lindenmeyer, Kriste. *The Greatest Generation Grows Up: American Childhood in the 1930s*. Chicago: Ivan R. Dee Publishers, 2012.

Luckingham, Bradford. *Minorities in Phoenix: A Profile of Mexican American, Chinese American, and African American Communities, 1860–1992*. Tucson: University of Arizona Press, 1994.

Marin, Christine. "Mexican Americans on the Home Front: Community Organizations in Arizona During World War II." *Perspectives in Mexican American Studies* 4 (1993): 75–91.

McLoughlin, Emmett. *People's Padre: An Autobiography*. Boston: Beacon Press, 1954.

Melton, Brad, and Dean Smith. *Arizona Goes to War: The Home Front and the Front Lines During World War II*. Tucson: University of Arizona Press, 2003.

Mendocino Beacon. Obituary of Ana Marie Bruenger. April 14, 2011. http://www.mendocinobeacon.com.

Mullenbach, Cheryl. *Double Victory: How African American Women Broke Race and Gender Barriers to Help Win World War II*. Chicago: Chicago Review Press, 2013.

National League for Nursing Education. *Standard Curriculum for Schools of Nursing*. Baltimore, MD: Waverly Press, 1917.

National Park Service. "Personal Justice Denied." January 8, 2007. http://www.nps.gov/parkhistory/online_books/ personal_justice_denied/intro.htm.

Pascoe, Peggy. *Relations of Rescue: The Search for Female Moral Authority in the American West, 1874–1939*. New York: Oxford University Press, 1990.

———. "Western Women at the Cultural Crossroads." In *Trails: Toward a New Western History*. Edited by Patricia Nelson Limerick, Clyde A. Milner II and Charles E. Rankin. Lawrence: University Press of Kansas, 1991, 40–58.

Payson Roundup. Obituary of Clara Rebecca Nourse Sumpter. December 13, 2011. http://www.paysonroundup.com/obituaries/2011/dec/13/becky-sumpter.

Phoenix Gazette. "Indian Service Family." March 7, 1945.

Pollitz, Phoebe, Carrie Streeter and Cynthia Walsh. "A Nurse's Journey." *Minority Nurse*, 2011. http://www.minoritynurse.com/article/nurses-journey.

Randolph, Pamela. "History of Regulation of Arizona Nursing Education." *Arizona State Board of Nursing Regulatory Journal* 6, no. 2 (2011): 6, 8.

"Religion: Too Material." *Time*, December 13, 1948. http://content.time.com/time.

Ridenour, Joey. "Arizona State Board of Nursing 1921–2011 90th Anniversary." *Arizona State Board of Nursing Regulatory Journal* 6, no. 2 (2011): 4.

Robinson, Thelma. *Nisei Cadet Nurse of World War II: Patriotism in Spite of Prejudice*. Boulder, CO: Black Swan Mill Press, 2005.

———. *Your Country Needs You: Cadet Nurses in World War II*. N.p.: Xlibris, 2009.

Robinson, Thelma, and Paulie Perry. *Cadet Nurse Stories: The Call for and Response of Women During World War II*. Indianapolis, IN: Center Nursing Publishing, 2001.

Roosevelt, Eleanor. "My Day." *Eleanor Roosevelt Papers Project*. Washington, D.C.: George Washington University, March 22, 1947. http://www.gwu.edu/~erpapers/myday/displaydoc.cfm?_y=1947&_f=md000606.

Saint Joseph's Hospital and Medical Center. *St. Joseph's: The First 100 Years.* Flagstaff, AZ: Heritage Publishers Inc., 1991.

Salsbury, Clarence, with Paul Hughes. *The Salsbury Story: A Medical Missionary's Lifetime of Public Service.* Tucson: University of Arizona Press, 1969.

Shields, Hazel, comp. *White Caps in the Desert: A History of Nursing in Arizona.* N.p.: Arizona State Nurses Association, 1969.

Staupers, Mabel Keaton. *No Time for Prejudice.* New York: MacMillan Company, 1961.

Summer, Mark. "The Real Greatest Generation." *Daily Kos.* http://www.dailykos.com/story/2007/10/14/397833/-The-Real-Greatest-Generation.

Thurston, Gorham, Thelma. "Negro Army Wives." *Crisis* 50, no. 1 (January 1943): 21–22.

Todd-Allard, Aleta. "Miracle on 7th Avenue: The History of Phoenix Memorial Hospital." *Today Magazine*, 1981: 10–16.

Towne, Douglas. "Health Before Habit: Father Emmett McLoughlin—Dubbed 'America's Most Famous Ex-Priest'—Was Chased Out of the Clergy After Founding the Valley's First Unsegregated Hospital." *Phoenix Magazine*, April 2013: 104, 106.

Trennert, Robert A. "Sage Memorial Hospital and the Nation's First All-Indian School of Nursing." *Journal of Arizona History* 44, no. 4 (2003): 353–74.

———. *White Man's Medicine: Government Doctors and the Navajo, 1863–1955.* Albuquerque: University of New Mexico Press, 1998.

U.S. House of Representatives. *Recruitment and Training of Nurses.* HR 2326, 78th Cong., 1st sess., H.R. 2326. Washington, D.C., 1943.

U.S. Public Health Service. *How Advertisers Can Cooperate with the U.S. Cadet Nurse Corps.* Washington, D.C.: General Printing Office, 1943.

———. *The United States Cadet Nurse Corps [1943–1948] and Other Federal Nurse Training Programs (PHS Publication 38).* Washington, D.C.: United States Government Printing Office, 1950.

U.S. Public Law 74. 78th Cong., 1st sess., July 1, 1943. Nurse Training Act of 1943.

U.S. Public Law 76-849, 76th Cong., 3rd sess., October 14, 1940. Lanham Act.

U.S. Public Law 93-203, 93rd Cong., 1st sess., December 28, 1973. Comprehensive Education and Training Act.

WETA and Latino Public Television. *Latino Americans.* 2013. http://www.pbs.org/latino-americans/en.

WNET. "Frances Payne Bolton, 14-Term Representative, Nursing Advocate." *Unsung Heroines: Celebrating the Accomplishments of Under-Recognized Women*. 2009. http://www.thirteen.org/unsungheroines/video/frances-payne-bolton-14-term-representative-nursing-advocate.

World War II from Space. TV movie, 88 min. London: October Films, 2012.

"The Younger Generation." *Time* 43, no. 19 (November 5, 1951): 45–52.

INDEX

D

E

F

G

H

I

J

K

L

M

N

ABOUT THE AUTHOR

Elsie Szecsy is an academic professional emerita at Arizona State University. She has an EdD in educational administration from Teachers College, Columbia University, a master's degree in comparative literature from New York University and a master's degree in secondary education from Hofstra University. Her undergraduate academic preparation is rooted in the liberal arts, where she began preparations for a career in teaching German, Spanish and English language arts.

Over the years, she alternated foci in her continuing education between educational topics—such as curriculum, instruction, educational leadership and educational administration—and humanities topics. Her studies in comparative literature served as a capstone to the multidisciplinary foci that she had developed over the years in languages and literature, cultural studies and the social sciences.

She is an experienced educator at the elementary, middle and high school levels. She also taught undergraduate and graduate-level courses on research methods in education, curriculum design and development, history and philosophy of education, educational assessment and educational technology. Dr. Szecsy administered a distance learning program, working with other administrators in a network of high schools across Long Island in sharing low enrollment courses.

In Arizona, Dr. Szecsy has been involved with a number of research and curriculum development projects in educational leadership and interdisciplinary studies, as both pertain to the unique U.S. desert Southwest–

northern Mexico region. She is most interested in educational projects that provide equitable access and outcomes in K-12 and higher education for all students, regardless of race, ethnicity, class or sexual orientation.

In retirement Dr. Szecsy mentors doctoral students in higher education administration, adult learning and educational leadership. Her independent research focuses primarily on cadet nurses' experiences.

When she is not researching or teaching, Dr. Szecsy enjoys knitting and gardening in her Tempe, Arizona home. She is also an avid walker, swimmer and bicyclist.